MEMORY LIVES ON
DOCUMENTING THE HIV/AIDS EPIDEMIC

Perspectives in Medical Humanities

Perspectives in Medical Humanities publishes peer reviewed scholarship produced or reviewed under the auspices of the University of California Medical Humanities Consortium, a multi-campus collaborative of faculty, students, and trainees in the humanities, medicine, and health sciences. Our series invites scholars from the humanities and health care professions to share narratives and analysis on health, healing, and the contexts of our beliefs and practices that impact biomedical inquiry.

General Editor

Brian Dolan, PhD, Professor, Department of Humanities and Social Sciences, University of California, San Francisco (UCSF)

Other Titles in this Series

Patient Poets: Illness from Inside Out
Marilyn Chandler McEntyre (Fall 2012)

Bioethics and Medical Issues in Literature
Mahala Yates Stripling (Fall 2013)

Heart Murmurs: What Patients Teach Their Doctors
Edited by Sharon Dobie, MD (Fall 2014)

Follow the Money: Funding Research in a Large Academic Health Center
Henry R. Bourne and Eric B. Vermillion (Spring 2016)

www.UCMedicalHumanitiesPress.com

This series is made possible by the generous support of the Dean of the School of Medicine at UCSF, the UCSF Library, and a Multicampus Research Program Grant from the University of California Office of the President. Grant ID MR-15-328363.

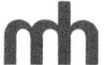

MEMORY LIVES ON
DOCUMENTING THE HIV/AIDS EPIDEMIC

Arthur J Ammann, Shan-Estelle Brown, Paul Burnett, Elizabeth Alice Clement, Lynne Gerber, Polina Ilieva, Jay A. Levy, Paul Volberding

© 2021 University of California Medical Humanities Press
University of California
Department of Humanities and Social Sciences
490 Illinois Street, Floor 7
San Francisco, CA 94143-0850

Cover Art: The NAMES Project AIDS Memorial Quilt panels displayed at San Francisco City Hall during San Francisco Lesbian and Gay Freedom Day Parade, 1988. Courtesy of UCSF Archives & Special Collections, AIDS Treatment News records, MSS 94-28, carton 41, folder 7.

Designed by Virtuoso Press

Library of Congress Control Number: 2021935883

ISBN: 978-1-6780-8982-5

Printed in USA

Contents

	Acknowledgments	vi
	Foreword *Paul Volberding, MD*	vii
	Introduction *Polina Ilieva, PhD*	1
1	The Importance of Basic Science in HIV/AIDS and Future Pandemics *Jay A. Levy, MD*	3
2	Contact Tracing/Partner Notification During the HIV/AIDS Epidemic *Arthur J. Ammann, MD*	25
3	Embedding HIV into the Undergraduate College Course *Shan-Estelle Brown, PhD*	49
4	Mobilizing the Oral History Archive: HIV/AIDS and the Multimedia Experience in the Classroom and Beyond *Paul Burnett, PhD*	67
5	Obituary Parlor Games: Collecting and Analyzing Obituaries as Sources for Understanding the AIDS Epidemic *Elizabeth Alice Clement, PhD*	76
6	Love is Stronger than Death: Making Meaning of AIDS in the Sermons of Jim Mitulski *Lynne Gerber, PhD*	96
	Index	106

Acknowledgments

The publication of this book was made possible through generous support by the National Endowment for the Humanities (Grant Number: PW-253755), UCSF AIDS Research Institute, UCSF Department of Humanities and Social Sciences, and individual donors.

Visit the UCSF AIDS History project website to learn more and access digitized collections: https://www.library.ucsf.edu/archives/aids/

Foreword

Paul Volberding, MD
University of California, San Francisco

From the HIV/AIDS epidemic's earliest days, those of us responding began to appreciate that what we were experiencing was somehow historic. The disease, AIDS, was certainly new. The cancers and infections we diagnosed were previously rare and without established treatments. The disease was uniformly fatal but often only after an agonizing collection of disfiguring and disabling conditions and months of inevitable disease progression. AIDS was visible; everyone could see the diagnosis. The public was afraid of AIDS, adding to the stigma already felt by many in the original "high risk groups", especially gay men and injection drug users. AIDS was quickly a political disease. The early governmental response was hesitant and in some instances hostile. At the same time, AIDS research was also exciting. It employed (and required) an array of new technology and knowledge of immunology exploded as a result.

The early response to the AIDS epidemic generated countless news reports but also an expanding collection of non-fictional works and memoirs. Reports including Randy Shilts' And the Band Played On, Laurie Garret's The Coming Plague, and Abraham Verghese's My Own Country were widely read and afforded valuable insights even as the epidemic was still evolving. The epidemic has also generated fictional work. In film, Philadelphia and Dallas Buyer's Club, and in theater Angels in America and Rent. But contemporary works have obvious limitations. Perspectives are often limited as are authors access to richer stores of information, much not available at the time to the public.

But histories of the HIV/AIDS epidemic will be written. Treatments now allow recovery from immune damage and have blocked transmission and new infections. The epidemic now feels mature, allowing a more stable and deeper perspective. Also, sources of information on the early epidemic response are becoming available. Archives of AIDS-related documents have been built and digitization facilitates access to data in a dramatically more democratic manner than previously possible.

As part of the University of California San Francisco Library, an ongoing creation of an HIV/AIDS archive is a vibrant project and is actively used in historical investigations. As part of the HIV/AIDS Archive, lectures and seminars focus on unique facets of the history of the epidemic response. The Archive organized and hosted a day-long seminar, including several lectures in this collection. They provide a glimpse into what we hope to gain from this continuing program. Authors range from a scientist himself involved in early AIDS research commenting on ways in which case contact tracing was (and often, wasn't) used to professional medical historians and educators. In one, fascinating insight into the social response to the epidemic is gleaned by careful reading of obituaries of AIDS deaths. This "obituary parlor game" shows ways in which the actual diagnosis was often disguised and the increasing recognition of the role of the same-sex partner of the patient in the common listing of survivors. Another paper in this collection explores the AIDS response in the San Francisco gay community through the collected sermons of an influential minister of a predominantly gay and lesbian congregation in the City's Castro neighborhood. These papers are clearly pieces of an incomplete puzzle but give us hope that as many others are added, we will gradually have the means of learning from an important collective experience. Since AIDS, we have seen yet more new epidemics including the searing and real-time disaster of COVID-19. We have much to learn form our response to HIV/AIDS and fully expect those lessons learned to help in the current pandemic and the others that will surely be visited on us. This collection is a very good start.

Introduction

Polina Ilieva, PhD
Archives & Special Collections, University of California, San Francisco

The AIDS epidemic has touched on all aspects of human life, political, socio-economic, cultural, and biomedical. For more than forty years all those affected by and those researching the epidemic: People Living with AIDS, activists, researchers, clinicians, journalists, historians, anthropologists, artists, and community organizers have been investigating and analyzing its impact on the society and ways to combat and eradicate it. However, these discussions have been siloed and those guided by the same aspirations rarely meet together. The goal of the **interdisciplinary symposium** *Memory Lives On: Documenting the HIV/AIDS Epidemic* that was organized by the UCSF Archives & Special Collections at the conclusion of a National Endowment for the Humanities funded project was to bring together these groups to explore and reflect on topics related to archives and the practice of documenting the stories of the HIV/AIDS epidemic. The Symposium program included a pre-conference workshop, six panel discussions on a variety of topics, and a poster session. Opening remarks were offered by Dr. Paul A. Volberding, UCSF Professor Emeritus of Medicine and Director of the UCSF AIDS Research Institute. Keynote addresses were made by Dr. Donald L. Abrams, UCSF Professor of Clinical Medicine; Dr. Jay A. Levy, UCSF Professor of Medicine; and Dr. Monica Gandhi, Director of UCSF-Gladstone Center for AIDS Research (CFAR), Associate Chief, Division of HIV, Infectious Diseases and Global Medicine, and Medical Director of "Ward 86" HIV Clinic at Zuckerberg San Francisco General Hospital. This symposium enabled historians, educators, artists, activists, clinicians and researchers studying HIV/AIDS in many different settings to share their work and experiences. The participants and attendees valued the opportunity to have candid conversations, make personal connections, and initiate joint projects. The majority of the sessions were recorded and these videos are posted on the UCSF Library website: https://lecture.ucsf.edu/ets/Catalog/Full/590301cfe126402ea81b329c7d113c2521.

This volume contains selected symposium presentations, due to the unfolding COVID-19 epidemic many presenters were not able to submit their articles and the editors hope that we will be able to expand and add new chapters as they become available.

The archivists strive to develop balanced collections that reflect views, decisions, and struggles of all sides affected by the HIV/AIDS epidemic. We recognize that our collections still have many silences and gaps, the voices of People Living with AIDS (PWA), many of whom were and are instrumental in bringing the attention of the medical establishment, government agencies, and general public to the AIDS crisis, are missing or underrepresented. Collaborating with these communities and individuals to collect and preserve their stories will enable us to create a more inclusive and equitable historical record. The UCSF Archives & Special Collections and other archival institutions are committed to serving as repositories of collective memory for all of those who experienced and continue to survive and fight the AIDS epidemic. The archivists continue to grapple with one of the major challenges - how to provide access to PWA stories in an ethical and respectful way without privacy violations, how to advocate and develop an inclusive and accurate historical record that binds together communal memories of patients, clinicians, caregivers, and researchers. The diverse documentary evidence that was brought to light as a result of this Symposium will enable the development of a complete and all-inclusive AIDS epidemic narrative where all those affected contribute their voices.

Chapter One

The Importance of Basic Science in HIV/AIDS and Future Pandemics

Jay A. Levy, MD
University of California, San Francisco

Thank you for the invitation to participate in this excellent symposium. I am very proud of my former students, Paul Volberding and Donald Abrams who are here and have been outstanding teachers and clinicians in the HIV/AIDS field. Today, I will emphasize my experiences in HIV/AIDS at UCSF. Everyone has their own version and I will be very frank, as requested by Polina, and share with you some history that is not well-known.

First, I would like to congratulate the UCSF Archives and Special Collections division and particularly David Uhrlich and Polina Ilieva for organizing this symposium. We hope the program will renew interest in those of you who look back at the issues surrounding HIV/AIDS and you will learn how to approach the next pandemic that comes to San Francisco. (Very prophetic since the symposium was held 3 months prior to the onset of the COVID–19 pandemic in San Francisco.)

For my topic, the title of my presentation states the obvious. During the onset and development of directions taken to handle HIV/AIDS, basic research played an important role – not only in the discovery of the virus, but also in the fundamental observations by academia that helped industry develop treatments and initiate approaches towards a vaccine. The latter, unfortunately, has not yet been achieved and is a notable challenge to our present and future biomedical research strategies. What I will share with you today are some of the important truths about the challenges faced by the initial group of UCSF researchers (basic scientists and clinicians as well as epidemiologists) who helped to uncover avenues that led to what I would say were great achievements in controlling this public-health challenge.

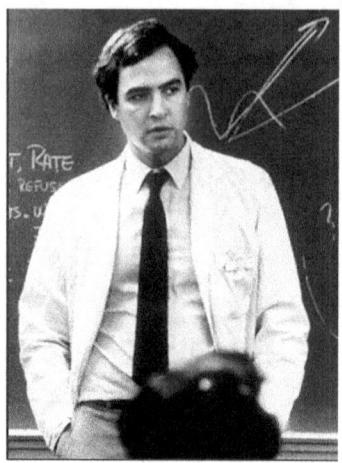

Figure 1: Paul Volberding

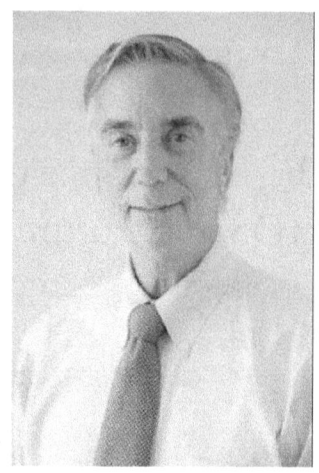

Figure 2: Donald Abrams

One of the first observations that I would make for those of you facing a new epidemic is the need to have financial support as well as the support from the administration. The environment is important for encouraging creativity, discovery and translation of science. Moreover, it is key to have a community that rallies to bring in subjects for study and to help develop programs that will lead to successful treatment and the needed government support—like NIH grants.

On August 6, 1981 I received a phone call in my office at the Parnassus campus. Paul Volberding was on the line. He said "Jay, I would like you to give a talk at San Francisco General Hospital (SFGH) Medical Grand Rounds next week. We have a young man with Kaposi's sarcoma (KS). With your known interest in cancer viruses, I would like you to discuss the possible cause of this disease. As you know KS is very unusual in young men and now KS is being seen in the young male population particularly gay men. It could be a virus. Donald Abrams is going to present the case." (Figs. 1 & 2) I immediately said yes and, at that meeting, discussed the possibility that a herpesvirus could be the cause. I had been in Uganda, Africa in the summer of 1964 as a medical student and had seen electron microscopic (EM) pictures of Kaposi's sarcoma tissues in which a herpesvirus could be recognized. At the time, we considered that this was herpes simplex virus and now, of course, it most likely was HHV-8 that was very much later discovered. (Chang et al., 1994)

In my SFGH presentation, I discussed why the herpesvirus seen by

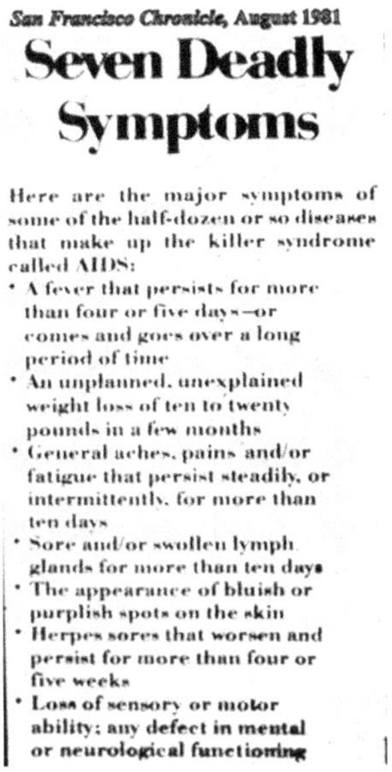

San Francisco Chronicle, August 1981
Seven Deadly Symptoms

Here are the major symptoms of some of the half-dozen or so diseases that make up the killer syndrome called AIDS:
* A fever that persists for more than four or five days—or comes and goes over a long period of time
* An unplanned, unexplained weight loss of ten to twenty pounds in a few months
* General aches, pains and/or fatigue that persist steadily, or intermittently, for more than ten days
* Sore and/or swollen lymph glands for more than ten days
* The appearance of bluish or purplish spots on the skin
* Herpes sores that worsen and persist for more than four or five weeks
* Loss of sensory or motor ability; any defect in mental or neurological functioning

Figure 3: *San Francisco Chronicle* newspaper article from August 1981 describing seven major symptoms of AIDS.

EM could not be the cause of this tumor but rather a virus that infected a growing tumor. My basic assumption was that if the virus is seen in a tumor, the tumor cells should be killed by its replication. My career had begun with an interest in latent viruses as a cause of cancer and, in that case, the virus would not replicate but remain restricted and perhaps produce a transforming protein. This SFGH conference was my first introduction to what had been called the Gay Related Immune Deficiency syndrome or GRID and KS was a major cancer in patients with GRID as well as lymphomas – both related to a disorder in the immune system (Levy and Ziegler., 1983). As noted in this newspaper article from the *San Francisco Chronicle* (Fig. 3), this new disease entity now known as AIDS looked like the flu or other common cold viral infections. It had symptoms of muscle aches, fatigue and what is most interesting at this very stage, symptoms of neurologic disease. (As an aside, it is also noteworthy that the coronavirus infection initially had an unappreciated effect on the brain most likely brought on by innate immune responses such as inflammation with coagulation defects.)

Donald introduced the patient, who later became a good friend of mine and the laboratory. He was 23 years old and had the onset of Kaposi's sarcoma a few months earlier. Following my discussion on the possible viral etiology of KS, I told Marc Conant, the patient's well-respected UCSF dermatologist and cancer doctor, that my lab would like to study his KS. We would see if we could isolate a possible causative virus. There was, however, a problem. My biosafety

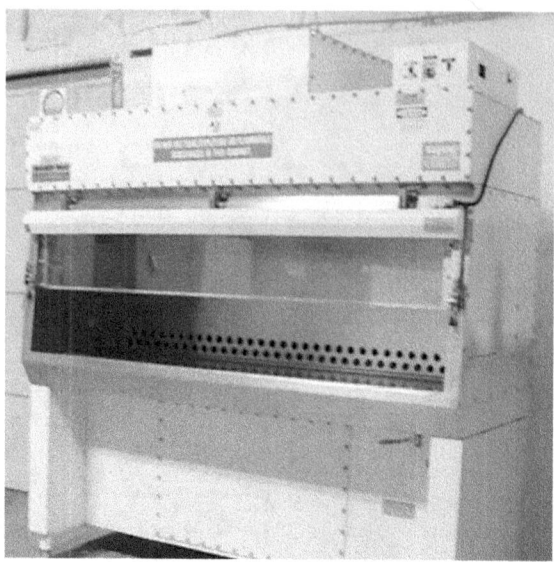

Figure 4: Biogard Biosafety Hood. The airflow is inward protecting the person working with infectious materials.

hood that I was using for mouse work was not, in 1982, at the correct safety standard for infectious human virus work (Fig. 4). I had to update it. This was my first financial challenge.

I needed quickly $1500 to get a filter for my biosafety hood. Therefore, I went to the UCSF Dean and asked "Is there a way by which I could get $1500 from the school to upgrade my biosafety hood? Then, I can begin my work on this new disease syndrome." He said "Jay, we really do not have the money for that. You should apply for a REAC (Research Evaluation Allocations Committee) grant for the funding." I replied, "But this disease is hitting our community now and it will take me at least nine months to obtain those funds. I would like to get started right away." The Dean said that, unfortunately, he could not offer any help.

Then, enters Marcus Conant who, during these early days of HIV/AIDS, was an unbelievable godfather to many people trying to find solutions to the new disease. Marcus said "Leave it up to me. Jay, I'll see what I can do." Then, it seems he went to the State legislature and they added a line item on a budget for "a biosafety hood for Jay Levy, $1500." Well I received that funding within 6 weeks. But I was then called to the Dean's office and "given the third degree."

"Why did you go around my back to get this money?" he asked. I responded, "Well, I couldn't do my work and Marcus Conant told me he might be able to help and he did." So I left the Dean's office thinking I am relieved that I can work but I feel now the space that will be needed to do the research probably will not be given to me by the Dean. That was another challenge I would later face.

At that time, in 1982, there was a KS clinic that Marcus Conant established at UCSF. It was an important addition to our study of AIDS. Every Thursday morning we would go to this clinic meeting in Mulberry Union on Parnassus Ave. Many clinicians and interested researchers were there as well as public health people including Selma Dritz and Andrew Moss. We learned from the KS clinic the epidemiology of this disease quite early after its onset. That information was exceedingly helpful as we considered the cause of the disease. We heard that the presumed infectious agent was passed by intimate sexual contact, blood and, later, by mother to child transmission. At first it seemed that GRID focused primarily on the gay community but soon the disease, known as AIDS, appeared in children, women and heterosexual couples.

One of the important issues raised at the KS clinic was, of course, what was the cause of AIDS? Marc had ongoing discussions, but one day the conclusion by some was that it could come from Haiti. That was because the Haitian population in Florida had a high prevalence of AIDS. Well, my sister Ellen Koenig lived in the Dominican Republic (DR) on Hispaniola, the same island as Haiti and I always visited the DR for the winter holidays. Therefore, in December 1982, I thought "I'll stop by Haiti on the way to the DR to search for a possible agent that causes AIDS." The one thought was African swine fever virus that induces immune deficiency in pigs. At that time, Jane Teas from London had suggested this idea later published in *The Lancet* (Teas, 1983) and received a lot of attention. Could that virus be the cause? So my wife Sharon and I went to Haiti and I looked for a possible animal reservoir. I found that, essentially, because of the poverty there, all the wild animals in the country had been killed. Only some chickens remained but that animal was not considered a carrier of a possible AIDS virus.

Nevertheless, when we were in Haiti we decided to see if there was something in a voodoo ceremony that might lead to passage of an infectious agent. Although only chickens were involved we paid a voodoo priest to hold a ceremony in December. Not surprisingly, there was nothing that suggested a way for the emergence of an infectious agent causing AIDS. Nevertheless, when I was in Haiti I was told that Port-au-Prince was a frequent holiday destination for the gay population in New York. Therefore, the virus could have come from NY. This could have been in 1978, four years prior to my visit to the country. Much later when we brought back HIV isolates from Haiti and compared them to viruses circulating in the United States, they were very similar in genetic sequence—both viral groups were Clade B. Of course, the virus could have come from Africa via Haiti and then to the States through New York. That possibility of transmission as early as 1978 has not been fully evaluated.

When I came back to California from my trip to Hispaniola, I gave a report to the KS clinic and we started asking again what could be the cause. Donald summarized some of the suggestions considered: intravenous drugs, seminal fluid, toxins, pollutants or a variant of a known virus. For the latter, Donald mentioned hepatitis B or CMV. Larry Drew liked the virus variant possibility and began looking for certain variants of known viruses in AIDS patients. My impression was that it had to be a new infectious agent and I felt that it would be a virus. This separation in effort looking for the cause of AIDS became a very cooperative venture for my lab and that of Larry Drew.

What was noteworthy about the UCSF experience, that I do not think was found elsewhere, was our aim to work together as a team. Nevertheless, as a reflection on one of my initial comments, we certainly did not have support from the administration. They did not want UCSF to be known as an AIDS University. They were afraid we would not get the best medical students, the best interns and residents so the aim was to keep our efforts "a secret." As a result, the few of us who were initially involved in GRID formed a tight unit working together. In this regard, there was a moment, early in our studies, that the Dean, at that time, called me to the office to tell me that he did not want to see any publicity on AIDS. This he said was not necessary and was not what UCSF should become known for. I remember being surprised and realized that Michelle Reichman, the UCSF Public relations director who was supportive of our work, had given us an opposite message. Her aim was to publicize the UCSF effort. The administration's view was unfortunate since we certainly would have received more financial support from the community at the time when funding was limited.

As is true for many health initiatives, funding for basic research studies was a major challenge especially for AIDS. In 1980, Ronald Reagan was elected the US President and one of the first things he did was to eliminate many grants from the NIH. He felt that industry and not government should take on that financial responsibility. All of my grants were cancelled and I did not know how I could obtain funding in a reasonable time. Fortunately, I knew Frank Rauscher from my NIH days in the late 1960s; he has a murine leukemia virus named after him. He was, at the time, President of the American Cancer Society. He gave me some funding (about $25,000) and through my Cancer

Research Institute colleague, Dr. Ellen Dirksen, I was encouraged to apply for a grant from the National Science Foundation. Ellen had a friend there and that helped. During these early days, I was then able to get, within a reasonable time, about $50,000 for my projects. This funding was needed to pay for salaries as well as supplies!

The money did help me hire students that could inject bloods from AIDS patients into a variety of animals to see if we could induce a disease. These consisted of small rodents such as mice, rats, guinea pigs, hamsters, and even ferrets. The bloods came from the AIDS Clinic at San Francisco General Hospital established by Paul Volberding. Paul was very helpful. Because the animals were injected with a possible AIDS virus, they had to be housed off-campus and were placed in a facility about 7 miles away in the same building in which Stan Prusiner had his animals for research on prions.

This financial need for AIDS research sparked the initiative of Paul Volberding and John Ziegler to submit a grant to the NIH in response to a request for proposals on AIDS that was advertised in early 1983. At the time, as I have said, Reagan was president and did not support studies of AIDS. He never mentioned the word AIDS in his first term of office. So here was a situation where the government was going to give a limited amount of money probably just to cover early efforts. We submitted the grant in February and received the funding in May. We had an excellent proposal that involved epidemiology, clinical work, and basic research. I recall that my culturing of KS cells from patients, such as Marc Conant's patient, was helpful since the NIH review committee recognized that we were already involved in looking for a causative agent.

In May, I also remember when receiving my funds that I had been given only $20,000/year for supplies. That seemed to indicate to me how NIH was not really expecting to have much done. I called the NIH administration officer and said, "I really cannot get much done with only $20,000 for supplies; please try to get me more money for our studies." He responded, "Jay, there's no more money. We just cannot give you more funds." "Well," I said, "What am I going to tell the journalists who call me when they know we are trying to find the cause of this disease. I can't get the government to help?" Two weeks later, I received $40,000 for supplies and that really made a difference.

At about the same time, in March 1983, the office of Willie Brown, the former mayor and, at the time, Speaker of the State of California House, called to say that the Speaker was looking to find funds for research in California to solve the AIDS problem. Thus, in May 1983, a group of us flew down to LA in the morning to meet at his office. This included Paul, John Greenspan,

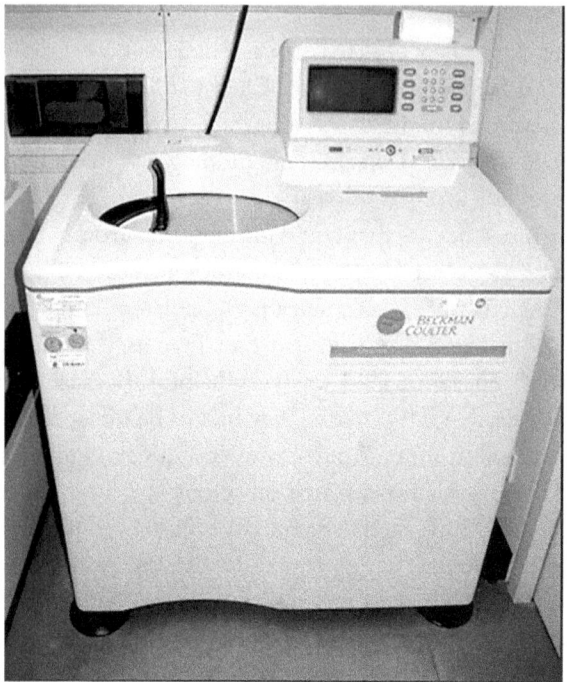

Figure 5: Ultra centrifuge used to obtain HIV from culture fluids.

John Ziegler, Art Ammann, Dan Stites, myself and from UC Davis, Murray Gardner. We boarded the same plane in San Francisco at 5:00 a.m. and arrived in Los Angeles early that morning. This visit is an important part of our history. And, again, another example of why it was important to not give up on basic science research studies.

When we walked into the Speaker's office, I was amazed to meet 6 secretaries waiting for us with electric typewriters (self-correcting!). They said, "We're going to get this grant written today." At this meeting, there were representatives from all the major schools in California including Stanford, USC and UCLA (that had a big effort towards AIDS). The Administrator in the office announced that I would be the head for the Virology group, Dan Stites for immunology, John Ziegler for clinical, and Paul Volberding for cancer.

Late that afternoon, we all came together with our different committees and turned in a budget that came to $2.9 million. At that time, $2.9 million was a lot of money. I was concerned and stood up and said, "This is a wonderful amount of money but maybe we should look again and not be so demanding. We could reduce the budget a bit." That idea never got appreciated: Everyone yelled out "Sit down, Levy."

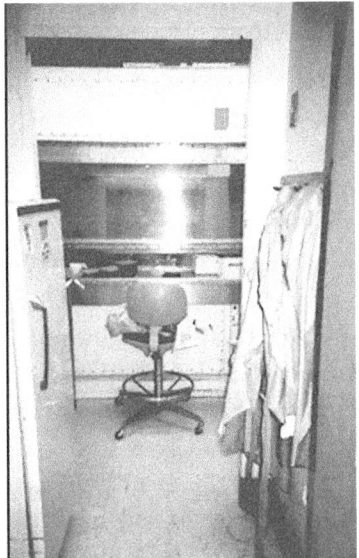

Fig. 6a

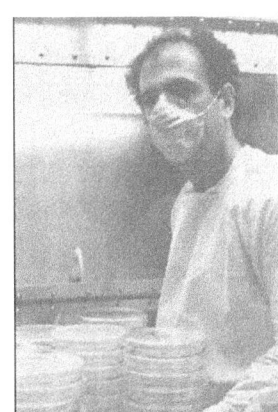

Fig. 6b

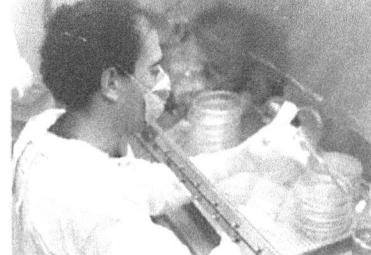

Fig. 6c

Figures 6a, b, c: (a) The Human Tumor Virus room S1269 in the Medical Sciences building at UCSF. A small outer chamber led through folding doors into a small laboratory with the biosafety hood and incubators. The author is visualized working with HIV specimens in 1983. This room and the materials inside are now at the Smithsonian Institute. Figures (b) and (c) show the author working in the lab.

Two months later, we received the total money, thanks to Willie Brown. Then, unfortunately, our Dean seized the funds. None of the deans at the other schools did this and their investigators got started on their studies immediately. Our Dean thought the grants were not given appropriate peer review. We all at UCSF tried to convince the Dean, the Associate Deans and others to release the money. It became obvious to us that the administration really did not want to support our efforts. Again, in relation to a theme of this talk, not having support for basic research studies from the University certainly hindered my early work as well as that of others. The Dean said that he was going to have a peer-review committee read our grant and he would release the money afterwards. What to do? It was clear then that it would be very difficult for a basic researcher as well as clinicians and other researchers to undertake a successful program.

In July 1983, I was invited to an international immunology meeting in

Kyoto, Japan where I heard the French scientists from the Pasteur Institute would be there. They had published in *Science* in April a study suggesting that the AIDS virus was related to HTLV. (Barre-Sinoussi et al., 1983) This conclusion was advanced because Bob Gallo at NIH had reviewed their *Science* manuscript and insisted that the authors describe their virus isolate as an HTLV - related virus. The French group, particularly Francois Clavel, spoke of their finding LAV—a retrovirus similar to HTLV in AIDS patients. I knew immediately that it could not be HTLV because that virus transforms human cells and does not kill them as this virus did, especially CD4+ cells, as was then known. In a way, this idea relates back to my SFGH Grand Rounds presentation in 1981. A transforming virus would not kill cells and AIDS patients were known to have a loss in immune cells. What was distracting was that Clavell at his talk said that they had only French bloods with antibodies to the agent. I thought that this was also not believable if true and felt that they really had an HTLV isolate only.

Afterwards, I flew to Paris for the wedding of my twin brother Stuart. Planning ahead I wrote to the Pasteur research group as we were all good friends. I had had a Sabbatical at the Pasteur Institute in 1979 with François Jacob and had done my virus work in the laboratory of Jean-Claude Chermann and later with Francoise Barré-Sinoussi in Luc Montagnier's group. Actually, I wrote to them early in April when their paper was published in *Science* and I congratulated them on their work. When I went to their lab meeting during my Paris visit in July I was then told that the virus that they found was killing cells so rapidly that they were not sure how they could easily keep it in culture. They said Clavel was misunderstood and that they really were finding antibodies in many different bloods. I realized then that Clavell had probably stated in English the fact that they had only really looked at French bloods for the antibodies. I mentioned this to Luc and Jean-Claude and said, "If indeed this virus is really the cause of AIDS, we should find it in our patients in San Francisco."

So, I went home and good news welcomed me. I had received the funding approval from the Dean to purchase the ultracentrifuge (at $50,000) (Fig. 5) we could now concentrate the fluids from our cell cultures from AIDS patients to see if a new virus was there. As you can imagine, I had tried very hard to borrow the use of a centrifuge, for instance, from Mike Bishop's group and others at UCSF but no one wanted the potential AIDS virus in their lab. Finally, at the end of September, I received the California State money from the Dean and purchased the centrifuge. We then had the following experience. In a very small 80 ft.^{2} lab, that had been modified for work with human cancer

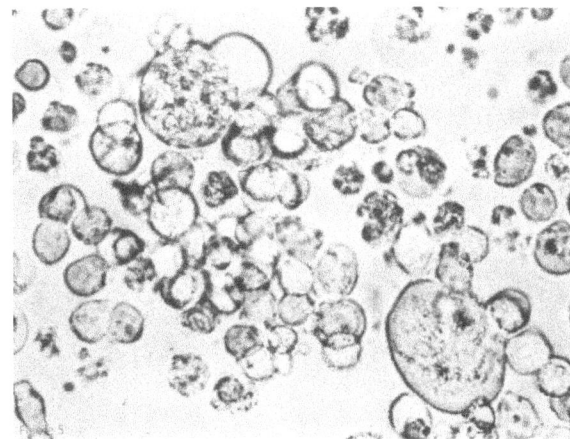

Figure 7: The typical cytopathic effects of HIV in cultured peripheral blood mononuclear cells. Note the balloon degeneration at the top right caused by inflow of sodium and potassium ions with water; at the bottom right is a large multi-nucleated cell X65.

viruses, we grew the white blood cells from AIDS patients. As is shown in Figure 6a, this lab had a small folding accordion door to separate the tiny entry where we took off our jackets and put on protective gowns. Then we opened the door and went into the small lab containing the biosafety hood (now updated for the study), an incubator, and a microscope.

We had in 1983 symptomatic patients coming from various regions in San Francisco, particularly Polk Street and then later Castro Avenue. Our procedure was to isolate the white cells from the blood of suspected AIDS patients and place them in culture. We separated these cells from the bloods from San Francisco patients including a classmate of mine from Wesleyan University. He had called me soon after I had arrived back from Europe saying, "I've got AIDS so maybe you can find something in my blood." We then put in culture his white cells coming from only 7 mL of blood as well as other blood samples from Paul's group at San Francisco General Hospital. Notably, in my Wesleyan colleague's cells, we saw these balloon shapes and multinuclear cells that were certainly not normal. (Fig. 7) We took the fluid from these cells and after filtering, added them to fresh normal white cells and saw the same effect. So we knew this effect was caused by a filtered agent, most likely a virus, and we needed to prove it. This was in October, 1983.

During this early research experience at UCSF, I had benefited a great deal from colleagues in virology that I had brought together in a group to meet on a regular basis. This gathering began in 1971 when I was working on mouse retroviruses. It included researchers from Berkeley, Stanford and the

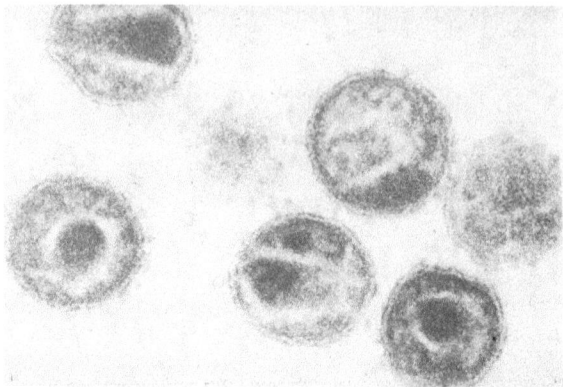

Figure 8: Scanning electron microscopic picture of the AIDS-associated retrovirus isolated in 1983. Photo provided by Lyndon Oshiro, San Francisco.

Bay Area dealing with what was then research with tumor viruses including retroviruses: Paul Arnstein, Howard Fieldsteel, Adeline Hackett, Young Kim, Walter Nelson-Reese, Lyndon Oshiro, John Riggs, Helene Smith, and Martha Stampfer. We would meet regularly and Walter suggested that we call ourselves "The Tumor and Virus Group of the West" or TuViGruWe! Therefore, when I thought we had this virus in the blood from AIDS patients I called up Lyndon Oshiro and I said "Lyndon, can you do EM studies for us as a coworker on the project." He said no problem, he would be happy to collaborate and this is what he found (Fig. 8). He had detected a retrovirus that had an eccentric nucleus. So, right away, we knew it was not HTLV but a lentivirus. It was a member of a different family than HTLV that then was known as an oncovirus. It took time for other research groups to realize this distinction.

Our paper on the AIDS-associated Retroviruses (ARV) was published in *Science* in August 1984 (Levy et al., 1984) three months after the HTLV-III studies were reported in *Science* by the NIH group. (Gallo et al., 1984) Notably, the three virus isolates: LAV, HTLV-III and ARV were suggested as a name for the virus. There was no consensus. I did hear that Donald came up with human immunodeficiency virus and also Robin Weiss. I had as well written it down but I knew by mentioning it, the name would not be selected. The field was very competitive! In any case, a committee did give the AIDS virus the official name, the Human immunodeficiency virus (HIV). (Coffin et al., 1986) And what the nomenclature committee also recommended is that each of the AIDS virus isolates should have a subscript giving the city from which the virus had been isolated. I, therefore, named our isolates SF for

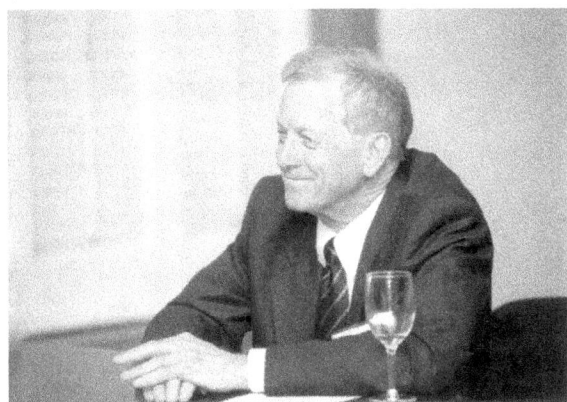

Fig 9: Bill Rutter

San Francisco and stopped counting at SF 147. Then when we found HIV-2 isolates, particularly from patients in the Ivory Coast, they were given the subscript UC for University of California. (Evans et al., 1988; Castro et al., 1990) (e.g., HIV-2$_{UC1}$)

So, having found what we assumed was the AIDS virus in San Francisco, I needed to do molecular work, especially cloning and defining its genetic sequence. We really were a biology lab and this aim was quite clearly a project in biochemistry. Therefore, I went to see a friend and mentor at UCSF, Bill Rutter, Chair of Biochemistry (Fig. 9), and said "Bill, I think I have isolated the AIDS virus and now need someone like you to help work with us. I cannot do the molecular studies in my lab, can you help?" Bill replied: "Jay, I can do it in my UCSF lab and work with you. "However," he said, "that could take 2 years. Why don't you look at my new company, Chiron, across the Bay and work with us there." I answered "Bill, in my training, especially at NIH, I was warned not to sell myself to industry. I cannot do that – my mentors would be upset and have a bad opinion of me." He responded "Well, just go look at my company and then decide. The company can do the cloning and sequencing in a few months."

So I went to Chiron and was "blown away" by all the equipment and impressive researchers I met. Thus, I came back to UCSF and said "Bill, my lab will be working with you." Subsequently, not only were we the first to clone the virus (Luciw et al., 1984) but also we were right there with other groups in sequencing it and determining its protein structure. (Sanchez-Pescador et al., 1985) Bill Rutter really helped especially with Paul Luciw and Dino Dina in his group. With their help and that of others we evaluated a large number

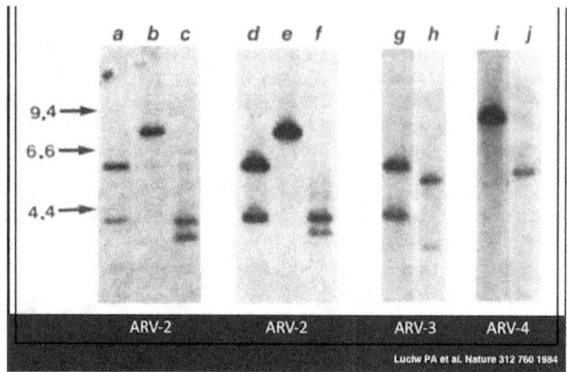

Figure 10: DNA Restriction enzyme pattern of four different AIDS associated retroviruses. Reprinted from Luciw et al.(1984) *Nature* with permission.

of isolates and determined their genomic nature. It was very early then that we recognized how different all the isolate were when examining the genome by restriction enzyme sensitivity. (Fig. 10) (Luciw et al, 1984; Levy et al 1985)

What also followed afterwards was an enormous amount of work done at UCSF on the virus, its proteins such as reverse transcriptase (RT) and many facets of AIDS. Several of the observations on the function of the viral proteins came from fundamental studies done a UCSF. Matija Peterlin's lab showed how the RT was very important in HIV transcription. (Kao et al, 1987) Later, Charlie Craik studied its protease that clips viral proteins into active enzymes. (Rose et al, 1995).

Then, in the summer of 1984, Murray Gardner called me and asked "Can you send me your AIDS virus isolate, ARV. I have received LAV and HTLV-III from Montagnier and Gallo and we want to compare their different genomes. Marty Bryant in my group will work on it. Subsequently, at UC Davis, they purified the viruses and performed the Southern blot analysis that confirmed our findings on heterogeneity. LAV and HTLV-III showed exactly the same viral genome. ARV was different. (Bryant et al., 1985) (Fig. 11) That raised a lot of eyebrows but the finding never really got a lot of attention. It was pretty obvious but the NIH group said that they never received LAV from Montagnier despite his saying that he had sent it several times to the NIH.

So now what happens? Why is there this virus heterogeneity? The explanation relates to the mutations that occur during HIV replication. When the virus infects cells and replicates, its reverse transcription enzyme (the one that makes a DNA copy from the RNA) is error-prone so it makes a lot of mistakes. Most of viruses formed are going to die but the ones that survive,

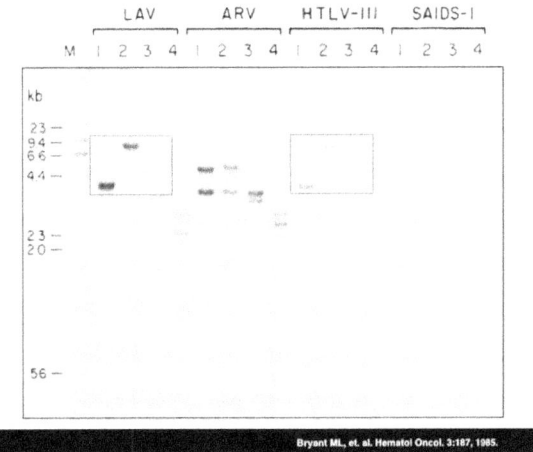

Figure 11: DNA restriction enzyme pattern of the 3 first HIV isolates and the simian AIDS D virus. Reprinted from Bryant et al. (1985) *Hemat. Oncol.* with permission.

replicate well and can become cytopathic or neuropathic going to the brain. In a sense, they are selected for their replicative ability (i.e., Survival of the Fittest).

So why was the finding that our ARV differed in sequence from the other two isolates important to basic research. That takes me to my visit to NIH in September, 1984. I was invited by the HIV/retrovirus group there to discuss my findings on the AIDS virus. I remember that Janet Hartley was at my talk. She had been a wonderful mentor for me at NIH, 1968 – 1970. During that NIH visit, Mal Martin requested that I stop by for a chat. I had known Mal from my time at the NIH so it was a nice reunion. After I had described our isolation of the AIDS virus and our antibody studies, he said to me "Jay, you need to be careful. I just came from a meeting at UC Davis and Murray Gardner's group presented evidence that indicated that LAV from Montagnier and HTLV-III from Gallo are very similar but your virus is totally different. That places your virus outside the general common characteristics of the other isolates. It seems to be a maverick." I quickly responded, "Well Mal, we have several isolates that were examined by Southern blot and they all are different. This information is being published in the *Annals of Internal Medicine*. (Levy et al., 1985)

At that moment, Mal gave out a cry that has become a legend in my AIDS presentations, "Oh my God," Mal said. Obviously, it became quickly evident to Mal that LAV and HTLV-III were the same virus. This fact was soon

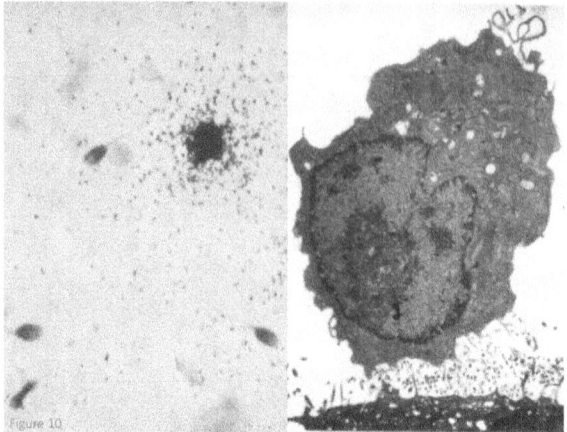

Figure 12: (left panel) Seminal fluid showing HIV infected cell with replicating virus detected by *in situ* hybridization; (right panel) HIV-infected cell interacting with cervical epithelial cells. Note the large number of virus particles at the interface. Reprinted from Levy (1988) *JAMA* with permission.

supported by several other observations such as the electron microscopic picture of HTLV-III published by Gallo that had been labeled on the photo in his lab, LAV. As noted above, while the Gallo group said they had not received LAV at any time, Montagnier claimed he had sent it at least five times. Now the proof was there. For some reason, I think politically, that information was never widely appreciated, stated or greatly considered. Some have said that it was hushed up by the NIH. Instead, Gallo and Montagnier, for some reason, signed an agreement stating that they found the virus at about the same time. The work of our group, without any receipt of a sample virus from the French, independently discovered the AIDS-associated retroviruses (ARV). However, our observations and our publication (just 3 months after the Gallo papers) were not well-cited. As I mentioned, competition was intense in this field. Our work continued and there were many examples told to me by individuals that NIH would take my name off invitations to conferences and one journal editor was threatened to not receive any submissions from the Gallo lab if it accepted my review on retroviruses. Fortunately, the paper was accepted and published anyway. (Levy, 1986)

In other research, our lab studied the basics of HIV transmission. We demonstrated that more HIV-infected cells were present in a seminal fluid than infectious virus. (Levy, 1988) (Fig.12) This observation remains an important fact for vaccine development. The finding argues strongly that there needs to be a strategy for vaccines to block the virus-infected cells. Moreover, we and others have shown that many different tissues can be infected by HIV. (Levy, 2006) Therefore, a cure needs to control or eliminate these cells. (Levy, 2015) That challenge is not well-appreciated by many in the scientific community who seem to believe that only the CD4+ T cell (and perhaps the macrophage) need attention.

Moreover, our early studies on the virus had important implications for hemophiliacs. Because the purification of clotting factors required chemical and physical treatments that I felt would inactivate a retrovirus. I called 5 different companies to see if we could spike plasma with the virus and determine if it survives or is inactivated by their clotting factor purification process. All the companies refused because of proprietary rights except one, Cutter Laboratories in Emeryville. Initially, they did not want to work with the AIDS virus so we gave them a mouse retrovirus, the xenotropic virus, that we could grow to a 10^8 titer. (Levy, 1978) This virus was put through the purification process by Cutter and the results were known in early March just before I attended a Gallo meeting at NIH on HTLV. The retrovirus survived the treatments and remained infectious without much loss of activity (Levy et al., 1984). That was one of the major reasons that we then rushed our paper to *Science*. I knew that I had followed the advice of my NIH mentors "to be sure of the implications of your findings before reporting the results."

It was now certain that HIV could be the cause of AIDS in all of the risk groups, including hemophiliacs. However, because of our waiting a few months, we missed the opportunity to publish before or at the same time as the Gallo group. Nevertheless, we had presented the evidence that this virus could survive Factor VIII purification and thus needed to be eliminated. The latter was achieved by a heating process developed at Cutter in which we showed that both the mouse virus and later the human virus could be inactivated in Factor preparations at 60° C without much loss of clotting activity. (Levy et al., 1984; Levy et al., 1985) We are, therefore, pleased that this focus on determining if the virus was the cause of AIDS in hemophiliacs led to a process of protecting many people from infection by clotting products.

One other example of the value of biomedical research as well as the collaboration at UCSF between researchers from different divisions, schools and disciplines is the study of oral hairy leukoplakia. That condition was discovered by Deborah and John Greenspan in the School of Dentistry. (Fig. 13) Working with them we showed the emergence of this unusual oral lesion as an early sign of immune deficiency in AIDS. (Greenspan, D. et al, 1987)

Let me end with a tribute to my early training with Gertrude and Werner Henle. They discovered that the Epstein-Barr virus (EBV) is the cause of

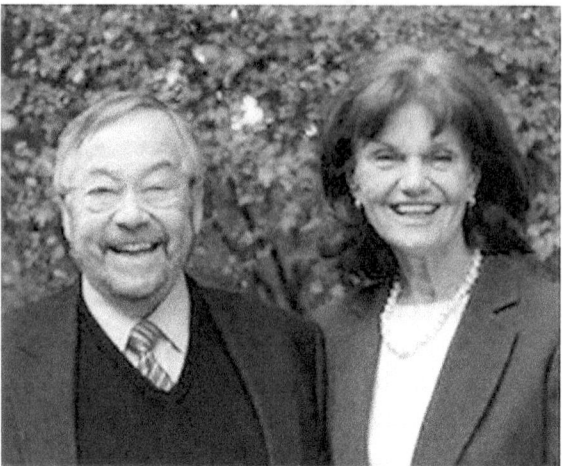

Figure 13: John Greenspan and Deborah Greenspan

infectious mononucleosis. (Henle et al., 1968) They taught me, during my internship days at the University of Pennsylvania, the immunofluorescence antibody (IFA) test. We used that procedure to show antibodies to EBV present in Burkitt lymphoma patients and normal children. The observation was made that higher antibody levels were found in the Burkitt lymphoma patients (Levy et al., 1966) and this finding led to the conclusion that immune enhancement could be playing a role in the development of lymphoma. This concept in oncology is popular today.

Then, in 1983, when we needed to look for antibodies to HIV, I developed an IFA test. I took Adi Gazdar's HUT 78 T cell line (Gazdar et al., 1980) (that the Gallo group renamed H9 without any attribution – see Rubenstein, 1990) and we established a HUT 78 T cell line in which every cell was infected. We then mixed that line with uninfected HUT 78 T cells so that 50% of the cells would show staining if serum antibodies to HIV were present. If all the cells stained, then autoantibodies could be involved and other tests needed to be done. Notably, that simple assay permitted us to detect antibodies within as few as 20 minutes when done by Larry Kaminsky, a Dermatology fellow rotating through my lab. (Kaminsky et al., 1985) (Fig. 14) He became an expert in undertaking these studies and also was testing blood from potential kidney transplant patients to rule out HIV infection in the donor. Our assay was also taught to Judy Wilbur at the State lab so they started using it before the Elisa became available in 1986. Evelyne Lennette at Virolab added the assay to all her antibody studies of children and adolescents as a service to clinicians.

Our most recent major focus in research is on an observation we made

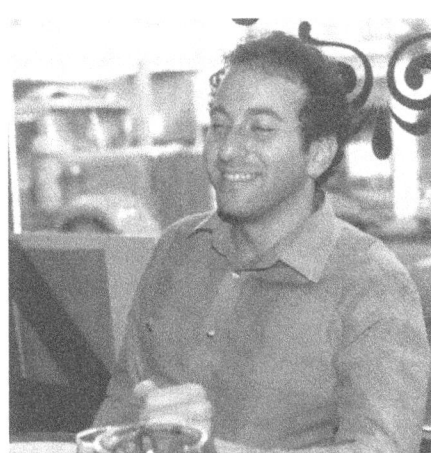

Figure 14: Larry Kaminsky

many years ago when we were isolating HIV from the white cells of suspected HIV-infected individuals. Chris Walker in my group found that, with the healthy infected individuals, the virus often could not be isolated unless we removed the CD8+ cells. The latter was accomplished at the time by panning (ironic for California!). (Walker, 1986) The CD8+ cells would stick to anti-CD8 antibodies adhered to the dish and the remaining cells were removed with the culture fluid. By this procedure, HIV replication took place in the CD8+ cell -depleted cells. The attached CD8+ cells, then recovered by washing the plate, were added back to the cultures. They inhibited the HIV production in the CD4+ cells without killing the cells. (Walker et al., 1986) When the CD8+ cells were again removed, the virus was produced; when the CD8+ cells were added back to the cells in culture, virus replication in the CD4+ cells was again inhibited. Subsequently, we found that the CD8+ cells produced a soluble factor, the CD8+ cell antiviral factor (CAF) which is associated with the inhibition of HIV replication. (Walker et al., 1989) We are still trying to define CAF which, as a low abundance protein, is very difficult to identify. (Levy, 2003) Notably, we had discovered with CAF a new mechanism for virus control by CD8+ cells: a non-cytotoxic antiviral response mediated by a soluble cytokine. This newly recognized antiviral activity has now been observed with other retroviruses as well as CD8+ cell anti-viral responses against herpesviruses and hepatitis viruses. (Levy, 2015) The identity of the CD8+ cell antiviral factor (CAF) is a continual focus in our laboratory. It is a natural immune factor that may play a role in other diseases such as cancer and autoimmunity.

In summary, we and others have made notable findings in basic science in approaches to combat the challenge of HIV/AIDS. We independently discovered the AIDS virus, helped to protect hemophiliacs from AIDS, and discovered a novel important non-cytotoxic CD8+ cell function in controlling viruses particularly HIV. In the search for CAF, the mediator of CNAR, the identification of other anti-HIV factors were discovered. (Levy, 2003) This antiviral factor merits identification and hopefully use in a therapy.

In this chapter, I have presented to you the exciting scientific, and somewhat difficult political, life of a basic researcher and the need for this approach in defining causes of new epidemics and microbe pathology. Our studies can lead to treatment and hopefully in the near future to a vaccine and cure of HIV infection. Certainly, support for basic science should continue to be a high priority as we go forth with the challenge of future microbial infections and pandemics (such as COVID-19).

Acknowledgments

The author would like to thank the support from the NIH, the Hellman Foundation, the A.M Dachs Foundation and the Campini Foundation. He also thanks his past research groups noted in the cited articles as well as the many patients participating in his studies.

References

Barre-Sinoussi, F., J.-C. Chermann, F. Rey, M.T. Nugeyre, S. Chamaret, J. Gruest, C. Dauguet, C. Axler-Blin, F. Vezinet-Brun, C. Rouzioux, W. Rozenbaum, and L. Montagnier. (1983). *Isolation of a T-lymphotropic retrovirus from a patient at risk for acquired immune deficiency syndrome* (AIDS). Science, 220, p. 868-871.

Bryant, M.L., J. Yamamoto, P. Luciw, R. Munn, P. Marx, J. Higgins, N. Pedersen, A. Levine, and M.B. Gardner. (1985). *Molecular comparison of retroviruses associated with human and simian AIDS*. Hematological Oncology, 3, p. 187-197.

Castro, B.A., S.W. Barnett, L.A. Evans, J. Moreau, K. Odehouri, and J.A. Levy. (1990). *Biologic heterogeneity of human immunodeficiency virus type 2 (HIV-2)*. Virology, 178, p. 527-534.

Chang, Y., E. Cesarman, M.S. Pessin, F. Lee, J. Culpepper, D.M. Knowles, and P.S. Moore. (1994). *Identification of herpesvirus-like DNA sequences in*

AIDS-associated Kaposi's sarcoma. Science, 266, p. 1865-1869.

Coffin, J., A. Haase, J.A. Levy, L. Montagnier, S. Oroszlan, N. Teich, H. Temin, K. Toyoshima, H. Varmus, P. Vogt, and R. Weiss. (1986). *Human immunodeficiency viruses [Letter].* Science, 232, p. 697.

Evans, L.A., J. Moreau, K. Odehouri, D. Seto, G. Thomson-Honnebier, H. Legg, A. Barboza, C. Cheng-Mayer, and J.A. Levy. (1988). *Simultaneous isolation of HIV-1 and HIV-2 from an AIDS patient.* Lancet, ii, p. 1389-1391.

Gallo, R.C., S.Z. Salahuddin, M. Popovic, G.M. Shearer, M. Kaplan, B.F. Haynes, T.J. Palker, R. Redfield, J. Oleske, and B. Safai. (1984). *Frequent detection and isolation of cytopathic retroviruses (HTLV-III) from patients with AIDS and at risk for AIDS.* Science, 224, p. 500-503.

Gazdar AF, Carney DN, Bunn PA, et al. (1980). *Mitogen requirements for the in vitro propagation of cutaneous T-cell lymphomas.* Blood, 55(3), p. 409-417.

Greenspan, D., J. S. Greenspan, N. G. Hearst, L.-Z. Pan, M.A. Conant, D.I Abrams, H. Hollander, and J.A. Levy (1987). *Relation of oral hairy leukoplakia to infection with HIV and the risk of developing AIDS.* J. Infect. Dis. 155: 475-481.

Henle G, Henle W, Diehl V. (1968). *Relation of Burkitt's tumor-associated herpes-type virus to infectious mononucleosis.* Proc Natl Acad Sci U S A, 59(1), p. 94-101.

Kaminsky, L.S., T. McHugh, D. Stites, P. Volberding, G. Henle, W. Henle, and J.A. Levy. (1985). *High prevalence of antibodies to AIDS-associated retroviruses (ARV) in acquired immune deficiency syndrome and related conditions and not in other disease states.* Proceedings of the National Academy of Sciences of the United States of America, 82, p. 5535-5539.

Kao, S-Y, Calman, A.F, Luciw, P.A, Peterlin, B.M. *Anti-termination of transcription within the long terminal repeat of HIV-1 by tat gene product.* Nature, 1987(330): p. 489-493.

Levy, J.A. (1978). *Xenotropic type C viruses.* Current Topics in Microbiology and Immunology, 79, p. 111-213.

Levy, J.A. (1986). *The Multifaceted Retrovirus.* Cancer Res. 46: 5457-5468.

Levy, J.A. (1988). *The transmission of AIDS: The case of the infected cell.* JAMA, 259, p. 3037-3038.

Levy, J.A. (2003). *The search for the CD8+ cell anti-HIV factor (CAF).* Trends in Immunology, 24(12), p. 628-632.

Levy, J.A (2006). *HIV Pathogenesis: Knowledge Gained after Two Decades of Research.* Adv Dent Res 19: 10-16.

Levy, J.A (2015). *Dispelling myths and focusing on notable concepts in HIV pathogenesis.* Trends in Molecular Medicine, 21: 341-353.

Levy, J.A. and G. Henle. (1966). *Indirect immunofluorescence tests with sera from African children and cultured Burkitt's lymphoma cells.* Journal of Bacteriology, 92, p. 275-276.

Levy, J.A. and J. Ziegler. (1983). *Acquired immune deficiency syndrome (AIDS) is an opportunistic infection and Kaposi's sarcoma results from secondary immune stimulation.* Lancet, ii, p. 78-81.

Levy, J.A., A.D. Hoffman, S.M. Kramer, J.A. Landis, J.M. Shimabukuro, and L.S. Oshiro. (1984). *Isolation of lymphocytopathic retroviruses from San Francisco patients with AIDS.* Science, 225(4664), p. 840-2.

Levy, J.A., L.S. Kaminsky, W.J.W. Morrow, K. Steimer, P. Luciw, D. Dina, J. Hoxie, and L. Oshiro. (1985). *Infection by the retrovirus associated with the acquired immunodeficiency syndrome.* Annals of Internal Medicine, 103, p. 694-699.

Levy, J.A., G. Mitra, and M.M. Mozen. (1984). *Recovery and inactivation of infectious retroviruses from factor VIII concentration.* Lancet, 2(8405), p. 722-3.

Levy, J.A., G.A. Mitra, M.F. Wong, and M.M. Mozen. (1985). *Inactivation by wet and dry heat procedures of AIDS-associated retrovirus (ARV) during factor VIII purification from plasma.* Lancet, I, p. 1456-1457.

Luciw, P.A., S.J. Potter, K. Steimer, D. Dina, and J.A. Levy. (1984). *Molecular cloning of AIDS-associated retrovirus.* Nature, 312(5996), p. 760-3.

Rose, J.R., Babe, L.M., Craik, C.S. (1995). *Defining the Level of Human Immunodeficiency Virus Type 1 (HIV-1) Protease Activity Required for HIV-1 Particle Maturation and Infectivity.* Journal of Virology, 69 (5), p. 2751-2758.

Rubinstein E. (1990). *The untold story of HUT78.* Science, 248(4962), p. 1499-1507.

Sanchez-Pescador, R., M.D. Power, P.J. Barr, K.S. Steimer, M.M. Stempien, S.L. Brown-Shimer, W.W. Gee, A. Renard, A. Randolph, J.A. Levy, D. Dina, and P.A. Luciw. (1985). *Nucleotide sequence and expression of an AIDS-associated retrovirus (ARV-2).* Science, 227, p. 484-492.

Teas J. (1983). *Could AIDS agent be a new variant of African swine fever virus.* Lancet, 321 (8330), p. 923.

Walker, C.M., D.J. Moody, D.P. Stites, and J.A. Levy. (1986). *CD8+ lymphocytes can control HIV infection in vitro by suppressing virus replication.* Science, 234, p. 1563-1566.

Walker, C.M. and J.A. Levy. (1989). *A diffusible lymphokine produced by CD8+ T lymphocytes suppresses HIV replication.* Immunology, 66, p. 628-630.

Chapter Two

Contact Tracing/Partner Notification During the HIV/AIDS Epidemic

Arthur J. Ammann, MD
University of California, San Francisco, Medical Center

Introduction

Contact tracing is a fundamental public health tool for the identification, diagnosis, and if available, the treatment of persons who may have come into contact with an individual infected with a transmissible agent. For sexually transmitted diseases, this is generally limited to sexual partners but for other highly transmissible infections such as Ebola virus, SARS, COVID-19 and tuberculosis information regarding casual contacts may also be required.

Contact tracing is essential for the control of the HIV pandemic. Since the HIV/AIDS epidemic was discovered in 1981 there have been an estimated 75 million individuals infected worldwide with 32 million deaths. Currently there are more than 1.7 million new infections and 800,000 deaths each year. Of the 38 million individuals worldwide who are living with HIV infection only 21 million are receiving treatment. More than 15 million individuals remain undiagnosed and unaware of their infection and therefore are untreated. (*Global HIV & AIDS statistics – 2019 fact sheet*, 2019)

The HIV epidemic continues to be firmly entrenched as a chronic global pandemic. In spite of major advances in identification, prevention and treatment of HIV international public health interventions have been inadequate to control the epidemic. Recent upsurges in the incidence of sexually-transmitted infections including syphilis, gonorrhea, and chlamydia add to the concerns that public health measures for controlling sexually-transmitted infections (STIs) are failing. The implementation of universal contact tracing for HIV, along with the strengthening of legal, educational, social, medical and community services, could bring the HIV epidemic under control.

History of contact tracing

Various approaches to contact tracing are likely to have been in place during many of the plagues throughout the history of medicine. Many of these were based on crude recognition of the external features of infection. As formal approaches to contact tracing were put into place, they were often misguided assigning blame to individuals who were minorities or lacked economic or political power. An early approach to contact tracing was put into place in 1864 following the approval of the Contagious Diseases Acts by the United Kingdom Parliament. The Acts allowed for compulsory registration and admission to the hospital of women judged by the police to be prostitutes. Women could be subjected to forced examinations for venereal disease (sexually-transmitted infections). Women who were judged to be infected were confined to a "lock" hospital until they recovered.

The first extensive use of contact tracing in the US occurred in 1938 under the leadership of Surgeon General Thomas Parran. (Parran, 1938a, 1938b) Parran was the first Commissioner of Health for the state of New York and the sixth Surgeon General of the US. He championed the National Venereal Disease Control Act which made funds available for rapid treatment centers that employed the new sulfa drugs and later penicillin. His public health approach to controlling STIs, which at that time was primarily syphilis, was outlined in his classic book *Shadow on the Land: Syphilis*. The principles that he promoted included a timely diagnosis and treatment of syphilis, screening for infection, partner notification, and public education and engagement. (Parran, 1937)

Although the public health principles established by Parran are credited with controlling syphilis the continued use of contact tracing for sexually-transmitted infections and other diseases often resulted in discrimination and violations of confidentiality. Parran himself was discredited for his participation in the infamous Tuskegee experiments that withheld treatment for syphilis from black men and failed to notify sexual partners of their risk of infection. (Park; Reverby) Nevertheless the use of contact tracing as a major public health tool for the prevention of infectious diseases is acknowledged as a fundamental public health tool for preventing widespread epidemics and pandemics.

Definitions

Contact tracing is the process of identifying persons who may have come into contact with an infected person and subsequent collection of further information about these contacts. Contact tracing may include referral to treatment. Partner notification also called partner care, is a subset of contact tracing aimed specifically at informing sexual partners of exposure to an infected person. ("Control and prevention of tuberculosis in the United Kingdom: code of practice 2000. Joint Tuberculosis Committee of the British Thoracic Society," 2000; "New guidelines on HIV testing and partner notification," 1992; "Partner notification," 1998; "Partner notification for preventing HIV infection," 1991; "Partner notification for preventing human immunodeficiency virus (HIV) infection—Colorado, Idaho, South Carolina, Virginia," 1988; "Public Health Service guidelines for counseling and antibody testing to prevent HIV infection and AIDS," 1987; "WHO Guidelines Approved by the Guidelines Review Committee. Guidelines on HIV Self-Testing and Partner Notification: Supplement to Consolidated Guidelines on HIV Testing Services. Geneva: World Health Organization," 2016) In this manuscript the term contact tracing includes partner notification.

Approaches to Contact Tracing

Partner notification is a principal public health tool for of controlling sexually transmitted infections and has traditionally been performed by public health professionals. After interviewing infected individuals, sexual partners are contacted and notified of the need for evaluation and treatment. The latter is known as provider referral, a relatively labor-intensive method. An alternative to provider referral is to have the infected individual conduct the notification (patient referral). The identity of the infected individual can remain confidential with the partner told only that they have been exposed to a specific infectious agent but not by whom. (Lunny & Shearer, 2011; Myers et al., 2003)

Innovations to contact tracing have increased the acceptability and success of partner notification. (Bernstein et al., 2014; Bilardi, Fairley, Hopkins, Hocking, Sze, et al., 2010; Bilardi, Fairley, Hopkins, Hocking, Temple-Smith, et al., 2010; Bourne et al., 2012; Carnicer-Pont et al., 2015; Cherutich et al., 2017; "Using the Internet for partner notification of sexually transmitted diseases—Los Angeles County, California, 2003," 2004) For example, coupling partner notification with expedited access to treatment or the use of the internet and social media to facilitate partner notification while protecting autonomy and privacy. Similar to the highly successful use of opt out HIV testing for pregnant women, opt out partner notification has increased the success of implementation programs. (Boer et al., 2011; Guy et al., 2013; Montoy et al., 2016) Studies showed that a low rate of acceptance was associated with an opt in approach (asking permission to conduct partner notification) compared to an opt out approach (stating that partner notification will be performed unless the patient disagreed). This significantly increased the number of individuals who agree to be tested. Simplifying consent for HIV testing is associated with an increase in HIV testing and case detection in highest risk groups. (Buchacz et al.)

Contact tracing for HIV

HIV is the only infectious disease causing a pandemic for which universal contact tracing has not been implemented. In order to understand this paradox an examination of the history contact tracing and the arguments against and for contact tracing is necessary (Tables 1 and 2 respectively).

When AIDS was first described in 1981 it was diagnosed by a set of laboratory and clinical criteria that defined the syndrome. There was no diagnostic test and therefore it was difficult to establish a precise diagnosis until advanced stages of the disease had been reached. Arguments against contact tracing emerged early in the AIDS epidemic. They emanated primarily from the gay community based on fears that the discrimination and stigma which many had already experienced might increase. (Lichtenstein, 2003) Additionally it was argued that since there were no drugs available to treat HIV (prior to 1987), the risks of HIV testing were greater than any potential benefit. (Gostin & Curran, 1987) Although calls for universal HIV testing in all health care settings were published as early as 1985, HIV testing was invariably disassociated with contact tracing.

In settings where HIV transmission was not sexual, contact tracing moved forward with little opposition. In 1984 the FDA approved an enzyme linked immunoassay (ELISA). It was immediately used for testing of blood donors to ensure safety of blood products. A rash of law suits against blood banks followed based on when blood banks should have known about possible HIV contamination of blood supplies and when they should have informed blood recipients that they had received "contaminated" blood. (Ammann et al., 1983; Ward et al., 1988) Contact tracing under these circumstances became mandatory. Initially it was thought that these lawsuits would accelerate the use of contact tracing for sexual transmission but sexual transmission of HIV

Table 1. Arguments against implementation of universal contact tracing for HIV

- Definitive diagnosis of AIDS is not possible (pre-discovery of HIV testing)
- No treatment is available (pre-discovery ZDV and HAART)
- Increases stigma and discrimination
- Loss of privacy
- Increases violence against women and marginalized groups
- Increases demand for prevention and treatment interventions that cannot be met
- Places a strain on already inadequate health care infrastructures
- Increases costs without comparable increased benefits
- Increases demand for healthcare professionals for prevention and treatment
- Weakens ethical standards of autonomy
- Weakens legal standards for confidentiality and privacy
- Fear of breaches in confidentiality may result in avoidance of care.
- Must remain voluntary

Table 2. Arguments in favor of implementation of universal contact tracing for HIV

- Required to define epidemiology
- Required for provision of life saving prevention and treatment
- Results in early diagnosis and treatment
- Identifies undiagnosed/untreated individuals
- Identifies other associated diseases (Tbc, STIs, GBV)
- Identifies new or existing areas of need
- Prevents late diagnosis and stigma associated with AIDS
- No documentation of widespread adverse impact
- Benefits significantly outweighs the risk of harm
- Accomplishes duty to warn/prevent harm
- Fulfills right to know/informed consent
- Brings resource benefits to individuals and community
- Affirms ethical principles of justice, equity, and beneficence
- Affirms individual right to health and life

remained as a protected sanctuary. ("Public Health Service guidelines for counseling and antibody testing to prevent HIV infection and AIDS," 1987)

In 1987 the US Public Health Service issued guidelines making HIV counseling and testing a priority for prevention and recommended routine testing of all individuals seeking treatment for STIs regardless of the health care setting. ("Public Health Service guidelines for counseling and antibody testing to prevent HIV infection and AIDS," 1987) The recommendations for voluntary HIV counseling and testing were expanded in 1993 to include hospitalized patients and individuals obtaining health care as outpatients in acute care hospital settings including emergency rooms. Both the initial and the expanded guidelines failed to recommend universal contact tracing.

The test of whether the availability of treatment for HIV would change HIV counseling and testing practices, including contact tracing, came in 1987 with the approval of the first antiretroviral drug, zidovudine, to treat HIV infection. (Fischl et al., 1987) Now that treatment was available, arguments were made that HIV testing and contact tracing should be routinely performed to identify large numbers of HIV infected individuals who could benefit from treatment. Nevertheless, issues of confidentially and discrimination prevailed and overrode arguments related to public health benefits. HIV became the only infectious disease pandemic for which prevention and treatment were available that did not call for universal contact tracing.

Moves to implement universal contact tracing should have followed clinical research reports at the 1996 International AIDS Conference in Vancouver documenting that early initiation of highly active antiretroviral therapy (HAART) dramatically decrease the progression of HIV to AIDS and associated mortality. (Detres, 1996; James, 1996; "Vancouver AIDS conference: special report. The epidemic now: current status and latest trends of HIV / AIDS in Africa -- a consensus update," 1996; Walters, 1996; Williams & De Cock, 1996) There were also reports that early treatment with highly active antiretroviral therapy (HAART) could prevent HIV transmission between sexual partners. The conference concluded with recommendations that HAART be initiated early in all HIV-infected individuals but recommendations fell short of calling for universal contact tracing to identify early HIV-infected individuals who could benefit from treatment.

An additional argument against contact tracing, especially among minorities and women, was that discrimination and gender-based violence (GBV) would follow notification of sexual partners. However, evidence for increased GBV following partner notification was largely anecdotal or failed to take into account the close linkage between HIV and GBV. In some studies

50% of women who suffered from GBV were found to be HIV-infected. (Decker et al., 2011; Dunkle & Decker, 2013; Forbes et al., 2008; Gielen et al., 2000; John et al., 2018; Koenig & Moore, 2000; Maher et al., 2000; Rosenfeld et al., 2016) HIV-infected men were highly likely to be engaged in GBV. Further HIV testing could be an entry point into identifying GBV, giving women legal rights and protection from violent partners and empowering women to obtain access and control of financial and other resources, enabling them to leave abusive relationships. (Koenig & Moore, 2000; Rothenberg & Paskey, 1995)

In the absence of contact tracing and partner notification a diagnosis of HIV may be time dependent. Without treatment HIV progresses to externally visible manifestations of AIDS. A suspicion or even a diagnosis of HIV infection by sexual partners can follow. Waiting until end stages of HIV infection creates greater difficulties in dealing with the diagnosis and managing healthcare. Delaying treatment for HIV infection by not conducting contact tracing complicates the management and care of an individual who has reached late stages of the disease and whose prognosis is significantly diminished. (Dixon-Mueller & Germain, 2007; Grinsztejn et al.; Ho, 1995; Lundgren et al., 2015; McDonald et al., 2006; Saag et al., 2018)

Studies on the outcomes of contact tracing universally report beneficial results. Name based reporting and partner notification following HIV testing in New York did not impact on the willingness to accept HIV testing among those at risk of acquiring HIV. ("New York issues draft rules for notification, surveillance," 1999; Tesoriero et al., 2008) The San Francisco Health Department received cooperation of both patients and named partners in notifying heterosexual partners of HIV-infected patients. (Buchacz et al.) In developing countries positive outcomes of disclosure for women include increased community and healthcare support, acceptance, kindness, and decreased anxiety. (Monroe-Wise et al., 2019; Omunakwe et al., 2015; Quinn et al., 2018)

Legal and Ethical Issues

In 2006 the CDC published new guidelines for HIV testing in the US. (Branson et al., 2006) While generally welcomed as a necessary public health measure for control of HIV infection, potential conflicts between public health and civil liberties were raised. Additional publications addressed the many ethical and legal issues that relate to HIV testing and their impact on confidentiality and discrimination. ("Ethical issues in the NIMH Collaborative HIV/STD Prevention Trial," 2007; Ewuoso, 2019; Fairchild & Bayer, 2011; Gibbs et al.,

2017; Golub & Indyk, 2006; Gruskin & Tarantola, 2001; "HIV Prevention Act would require HIV reporting," 1997; "Is partner notification in the public interest?," 1999; Lamboi & Sy, 1989; Levine, 1988; Onotai et al., 2004)

There is recognition that that there is both a legal and ethical requirement to prevent the transmission of HIV. (Cason et al., 2002; Clark, 1990; Gostin & Curran, 1986, 1987; Gruskin & Tarantola, 2001; Lamboi & Sy, 1989; O'Brien, 1993) Blood testing of blood donors is accepted as necessary and legally required. (Ward et al., 1988) If an individual receives a blood product that is identified as having been obtained from an HIV infected individual there is a legal and ethical duty to warn and to perform contact tracing. Differences between legal and ethical requirements are primarily based on the mode of transmission e.g. differentiation of transmission by blood or transmission by sex is not supported by public health principles.

Legal guidelines related to contact tracing and disclosure may very under state law. Under the Illinois Confidentiality of HIV-Related Information Act, a physician may disclose confidential HIV-related information to a known contact of the patient. (Health, 2015) A California appeals court concluded that physicians have an obligation to tell infected patients that they have a contagious disease so that patients and people around them can avoid spreading the illness. Courts in other states have ruled differently contributing to a lack of clarity in ethical and legal obligations and the principle of a duty to inform.

Proponents of contact tracing often refer to the duty of a healthcare professional to inform an individual of a potential hazard. This has been largely driven by the landmark case of *Tarasoff vs the Regents of the University of California*. In a majority opinion, California's Supreme Court ruled that medical confidentiality must yield to public interest in safety from violent assault. (Binder & McNiel, 1996; Walcott et al., 2001) In Tarasoff, a psychologist failed to warn a woman or her family of a threat that a patient made to murder a woman. In spite of the California Supreme Court decision the principle of duty to inform has been only theoretically applied to the transmission of HIV except in instances where the transmission has been deliberate. (Ketels & Vander Beken, 2012; Nie et al., 2015; O'Brien, 1993; Rose, 2001) Mandatory contact tracing for HIV in New York was triggered after 10 women were infected with HIV by one man in NY state. The law was based on the need to identify additional individuals who might be HIV infected and require treatment. ("Cluster of HIV-positive young women--New York, 1997-1998," 1999)

An early worrisome trend associated with name reporting of HIV infection were attempts to criminalizing HIV transmission. These were misguided attempts to stigmatize HIV infected individuals. Early passage of legislation in the US, Africa, and European countries were eventually dismissed or were left unenforced. (Arreola et al., 2015; Burris & Cameron, 2008; Cameron, 2009; Mayer et al., 2018; Patterson et al., 2015)

International laws that apply to rape as crimes against humanity are in place when rape is employed, usually by rebel troops, as a deliberate means of demoralizing individuals and communities. WHO formally recognized the use of rape against women during war as a crime against humanity but not deliberate HIV infection. During the Rwandan genocide many of the rebel soldiers were aware that rape coupled with HIV infection could inflect harm on women, their families, communities, and future generations of children. (Donovan, 2002) Rape along with transmission of HIV and other STIs continues as a means of warfare in Eastern Congo. (Brown; Kabengele Mpinga et al.)

Legal and ethical concepts have been widely discussed in relationship to voluntary versus mandatory contact tracing. (Bayer, 1989; Bayer & Toomey, 1992; Chervenak et al., 1997; Hildesheimer, 2002; "WHO Guidelines Approved by the Guidelines Review Committee," 2016) Strict interpretation of autonomy and confidentiality are employed as reasons for not conducting contact tracing. Autonomy along with confidentiality is interpreted to mean that only an individual can determine whether or not contact tracing can be performed in spite of potential public good. The introduction of Western based concepts of autonomy and confidentially into cultures that rely on family and community based support for survival, in the absence of the strong health and legal infrastructure in developed countries, has been questioned. (Epstein, 2007) Western views of confidentiality hold that a physician-patient relationship of trust requires respect for confidentiality and that a physician has a professional obligation to uphold a patient's expectations of privacy. (Epstein, 2007; Farmer, 1999)

In resource poor settings, confidentiality without access to health care can result in denial of health care to the most vulnerable populations, primarily women and children including those with advanced stages of HIV infection. Women in resource poor settings, who are often politically and socially powerless often view confidential HIV testing as a means of allowing men to continue to practice unprotected sex and exert their dominance over women.

While there are many arguments for maintaining confidentiality there are instances where confidentiality may be broken, and in fact there are circumstances where a physician is obligated to break confidentiality. Laws are in place in many states in the US that require physicians to report specific infectious diseases including STIs to public health authorities in order to protect the health of the community. ("Cluster of HIV-positive young women—New York, 1997-1998," 1999) Similar laws hold that healthcare professionals are required to report suspected child abuse in a minor, instances of GBV and protection of blood donor recipients from infected blood products. (English, 2017; Liu & Vaughn; Rodríguez et al., 2001)

Contact tracing for HIV and other STIs

Historically, contact tracing was first formally implemented for the control of syphilis. (Parran, 1937) A groundbreaking approach was championed by Parran in 1938 which establish the fundamental principles of contact tracing — a timely diagnosis and treatment, screening for infection, partner notification, and public education and engagement.. As a result, the syphilis epidemic in the US came under control.

In the early 2000s reports began to appear that there were increases of sexually-transmitted infections in HIV-infected individuals. (Gunn et al., 1995; Kerani et al., 2007; Kissinger et al., 2003; Peterman et al., 2015; Polansky et al., 2019; Tan et al., 2016; Thomas et al., 2016) As HIV is also a sexually transmitted infection it was not a surprise to some that syphilis, gonorrhea, and chlamydia might make a reappearance in HIV infected individuals after decades of control. Reports observed that an increase in HIV infection in men who have sex with men was associated with a tenfold increase in primary and secondary syphilis. New cases of chlamydia, gonorrhea, and syphilis rose sharply in 2017 to a record high of 2.3 million. There were also reports that HIV infection increased as much as a fivefold in the presence of other STIs. Syphilis rates were two times higher in African-Americans than whites. (Bradley et al.; "Epidemic early syphilis—Montgomery County, Alabama, 1990-1991," 1992; "Outbreak of primary and secondary syphilis—Baltimore City, Maryland, 1995," 1996; "Primary and secondary syphilis—Jefferson county, Alabama, 2002-2007," 2009)

An explanation for the rise in STIs in HIV-infected individuals was that individuals lacked an awareness of their HIV infection and therefore continued high risk behaviors thereby increasing exposure to STIs. (Hampton, 2008) An alternative explanation might be that this is an acknowledgment that the public health approach for the control of STIs has faltered as a result of a diminished emphasis on contact tracing for HIV. Testing for STIs requires inclusion of all sexually transmitted infections including HIV and the incorporation of contact tracing to identify individuals in need of prevention and treatment. In addition to reports of increased co-infections with syphilis and HIV in men and women there were reports that congenital syphilis, long felt to be under control, is increasing. (Plotzker et al., 2018; Rubin)

Social and cultural considerations

Contact tracing must also take into account the sociology and cultural aspects of the society in which an HIV epidemic occurs. (Epstein, 2007; Sovran, 2013) Some sociologists have suggested that the US and Europe have exerted undue influence on developing countries in relation to HIV testing and contract tracing as a result of a strong shift in their countries to individual rights. Insistence on Western principles of confidentiality and contact tracing are felt to be a means of enforcing male dominance resulting in violation of a woman's right to health and life. During the time of delayed diagnosis, the right of a woman to treatment is denied, and if she becomes pregnant, her right to protect her infant from HIV infection is also denied.

Alternatively, it could be argued that the failure to perform universal HIV testing and to require partner notification denies civil liberties to a majority of those in the HIV epidemic, especially women, the poor, and marginalized individuals, who require special protection and advocacy. Without knowledge of a sexual partner's HIV status, individuals are denied the right to protect themselves from a fatal HIV infection or if already infected, denied access to potentially lifesaving interventions. The continued marked discrepancy in HIV infection rates and access to prevention and treatment in both the US and in resource poor countries in the poor, people of color, women, and marginalized populations suggests an indifference to the health of these populations. Identification of individuals who have been exposed to HIV, or who are already infected, by means of contact tracing would provide them with lifesaving prevention and treatment. Failure to do so suggests underlying discriminatory and misogynistic attitudes in public health implementation. (Cargill & Stone, 2005; Essuon et al., 2020; Hyman et al., 1999; Kanny et al.; Laurencin et al., 2008; Magadi, 2013; Reif et al., 2014; Stone, 2012)

Summary

More than 40 years after AIDS was first described it is apparent that there has been a global public health failure to control the HIV pandemic. Contact tracing, long a fundamental tool for the control of infectious

> **Table 3. Possible future adverse outcomes of failing to implement universal contact tracing**
>
> - Inability to achieve international health organization goals for control of HIV
> - Over the next five years 10 million new HIV infections and 5 million additional HIV-infected individuals unable to access treatment
> - Loss of healthcare resources as a result of economic competition
> - Increasing discrimination against disadvantaged and marginalized populations
> - Increased numbers of co-infections with STIs and opportunistic infections
> - Emergence of multiple drug resistant HIV
> - Unaffordability of new treatments as HIV drug resistance increases
> - Economic competition of HIV with other acute and chronic diseases
> - Selective denial of life saving prevention treatment to vulnerable populations
> - Increasing conflict between individual rights and public health obligations

disease epidemics, has been a neglected intervention for bringing the HIV pandemic under control. Initial opposition to contact tracing and partner notification was justified on the basis of legal and ethical principles to protect the autonomy and privacy of individuals and to prevent the discrimination, stigma and violence associated with a diagnosis of HIV or AIDS. Many of these obstacles have been overcome in resource rich countries that have well-established legal, ethical, and political means of protection and where individuals can gain access to lifesaving prevention and treatment. However, both in resource poor countries, and in resource poor settings in the US, many disadvantaged individuals lack these same protections. It is likely that the continued failure to implement universal contact tracing will be associated with substantial adverse outcomes. (Table 3) A general indifference to the millions of new infections and deaths will sustain the HIV pandemic in spite of the remarkable prevention and treatment approaches that are available. As millions of additional individuals become infected annually, all requiring treatment, the burden on healthcare infrastructure in resource poor countries will not accommodate the cost of maintaining individuals on lifelong treatment. Increasing drug resistance will shift prevention and treatment to more expensive and less available approaches, placing strains on healthcare priorities. The continued omission of universal contact tracing from the global health prevention and treatment armamentarium can no longer be justified ethically or by public health principles. Without a dramatic expansion of contact tracing millions of individuals remain excluded from lifesaving HIV prevention and treatment measures. The majority of these individuals will be susceptible to discrimination and marginalization. Universal opt out contact tracing is a necessary means of implementing lifesaving measures for bringing the HIV/AIDS epidemic under control.

References

Ammann, A. J., Cowan, M. J., Wara, D. W., Weintrub, P., Dritz, S., Goldman, H., & Perkins, H. A. (1983, Apr 30). Acquired immunodeficiency in an infant: possible transmission by means of blood products. *Lancet, 1*(8331), 956-958. https://doi.org/10.1016/s0140-6736(83)92082-2

Arreola, S., Santos, G. M., Beck, J., Sundararaj, M., Wilson, P. A., Hebert, P., Makofane, K., Do, T. D., & Ayala, G. (2015, Feb). Sexual stigma, criminalization, investment, and access to HIV services among men who have sex with men worldwide. *AIDS Behav, 19*(2), 227-234. https://doi.org/10.1007/s10461-014-0869-x

Bayer, R. (1989, Mar). Ethical and social policy issues raised by HIV screening: the epidemic evolves and so do the challenges. *Aids, 3*(3), 119-124. https://doi.org/10.1097/00002030-198903000-00001

Bayer, R., & Toomey, K. E. (1992, Aug). HIV prevention and the two faces of partner notification. *Am J Public Health, 82*(8), 1158-1164. https://doi.org/10.2105/ajph.82.8.1158

Bernstein, K. T., Stephens, S. C., Moss, N., Scheer, S., Parisi, M. K., & Philip, S. S. (2014, Jan-Feb). Partner services as targeted HIV screening--changing the paradigm. *Public Health Rep, 129 Suppl 1*, 50-55. https://doi.org/10.1177/00333549141291s108

Bilardi, J. E., Fairley, C. K., Hopkins, C. A., Hocking, J. S., Sze, J. K., & Chen, M. Y. (2010, Sep). Let Them Know: evaluation of an online partner notification service for chlamydia that offers E-mail and SMS messaging. *Sex Transm Dis, 37*(9), 563-565. https://doi.org/10.1097/OLQ.0b013e3181d707f1

Bilardi, J. E., Fairley, C. K., Hopkins, C. A., Hocking, J. S., Temple-Smith, M.

J., Bowden, F. J., Russell, D. B., Pitts, M., Tomnay, J. E., Parker, R. M., Pavlin, N. L., & Chen, M. Y. (2010, Apr). Experiences and outcomes of partner notification among men and women recently diagnosed with Chlamydia and their views on innovative resources aimed at improving notification rates. *Sex Transm Dis, 37*(4), 253-258. https://doi.org/10.1097/OLQ.0b013e3181d012e0

Binder, R. L., & McNiel, D. E. (1996, Nov). Application of the Tarasoff ruling and its effect on the victim and the therapeutic relationship. *Psychiatr Serv, 47*(11), 1212-1215.

Boer, K., Smit, C., van der Flier, M., & de Wolf, F. (2011, Oct). The comparison of the performance of two screening strategies identifying newly-diagnosed HIV during pregnancy. *Eur J Public Health, 21*(5), 632-637. https://doi.org/10.1093/eurpub/ckq157

Bourne, C., Zablotska, I., Williamson, A., Calmette, Y., & Guy, R. (2012, Sep). Promotion and uptake of a new online partner notification and retesting reminder service for gay men. *Sex Health, 9*(4), 360-367. https://doi.org/10.1071/sh11132

Bradley, E. L. P., Williams, A. M., Green, S., Lima, A. C., Geter, A., Chesson, H. W., & McCree, D. H. (May 10). Disparities in Incidence of Human Immunodeficiency Virus Infection Among Black and White Women - United States, 2010-2016. *MMWR Morb Mortal Wkly Rep, 68*(18), 416-418.

Branson, B. M., Handsfield, H. H., Lampe, M. A., Janssen, R. S., Taylor, A. W., Lyss, S. B., & Clark, J. E. (2006, Sep 22). Revised recommendations for HIV testing of adults, adolescents, and pregnant women in health-care settings. *MMWR Recomm Rep, 55*(Rr-14), 1-17; quiz CE11-14.

Brown, C. Rape as a weapon of war in the Democratic Republic of the Congo. *Torture, 22*(1), 24-37.

Buchacz, K., Chen, M. J., Parisi, M. K., Yoshida-Cervantes, M., Antunez, E., Delgado, V., Moss, N. J., & Scheer, S. Using HIV surveillance registry data to re-link persons to care: the RSVP Project in San Francisco. *PLoS One, 10*(3), e0118923.

Burris, S., & Cameron, E. (2008, Aug 6). The case against criminalization of HIV transmission. *Jama, 300*(5), 578-581. https://doi.org/10.1001/jama.300.5.578

Cameron, E. (2009, Dec). Criminalization of HIV transmission: poor public health policy. *HIV AIDS Policy Law Rev, 14*(2), 1, 63-75.

Cargill, V. A., & Stone, V. E. (2005, Jul). HIV/AIDS: a minority health issue. *Med Clin North Am, 89*(4), 895-912. https://doi.org/10.1016/j.mcna.2005.03.005

Carnicer-Pont, D., Barbera-Gracia, M. J., Fernandez-Davila, P., Garcia de Olalla, P., Munoz, R., Jacques-Avino, C., Saladie-Marti, M. P., Gosch-Elcoso, M., Arellano Munoz, E., & Casabona, J. (2015, May-Jun). Use of new technologies to notify possible contagion of sexually-transmitted infections among men. *Gac Sanit, 29*(3), 190-197. https://doi.org/10.1016/j.gaceta.2015.01.003

Cason, C., Orrock, N., Schmitt, K., Tesoriero, J., Lazzarini, Z., & Sumartojo, E. (2002, Fall). The impact of laws on HIV and STD prevention. *J Law Med Ethics, 30*(3 Suppl), 139-145.

Cherutich, P., Golden, M. R., Wamuti, B., Richardson, B. A., Asbjornsdottir, K. H., Otieno, F. A., Ng'ang'a, A., Mutiti, P. M., Macharia, P., Sambai, B., Dunbar, M., Bukusi, D., & Farquhar, C. (2017, Feb). Assisted partner services for HIV in Kenya: a cluster randomised controlled trial. *Lancet HIV, 4*(2), e74-e82. https://doi.org/10.1016/s2352-3018(16)30214-4

Chervenak, F. A., McCullough, L. B., & Ledger, W. J. (1997). Ethical dimensions of human immunodeficiency virus infection during pregnancy. *Infect Dis Obstet Gynecol, 5*(2), 192-198. https://doi.org/10.1155/s106474499700029x

Clark, M. E. (1990). AIDS prevention: legislative options. *Am J Law Med, 16*(1-2), 107-153.

Cluster of HIV-positive young women--New York, 1997-1998. (1999, May 28). *MMWR Morb Mortal Wkly Rep, 48*(20), 413-416.

Control and prevention of tuberculosis in the United Kingdom: code of practice 2000. Joint Tuberculosis Committee of the British Thoracic Society. (2000, Nov). *Thorax, 55*(11), 887-901. https://doi.org/10.1136/thorax.55.11.887

Decker, M. R., Miller, E., McCauley, H. L., Tancredi, D. J., Levenson, R. R., Waldman, J., Schoenwald, P., & Silverman, J. G. (2011, Jun). Intimate partner violence and partner notification of sexually transmitted infections among adolescent and young adult family planning clinic patients. *Int J STD AIDS, 22*(6), 345-347. https://doi.org/10.1258/ijsa.2011.010425

Detres, L. L. (1996, Oct-Nov). [The new age of HIV/AIDS. A special report on the XI International Conference on AIDS]. *Sidahora*, 26-33. (La nueva era del VIH/SIDA. Reporte especial sobre la XI Conferencia Internacional del SIDA.)

Dixon-Mueller, R., & Germain, A. (2007, Dec 1). HIV testing: the mutual rights and responsibilities of partners. *Lancet, 370*(9602), 1808-1809.

Donovan, P. (2002, Dec). Rape and HIV/AIDS in Rwanda. *Lancet, 360 Suppl*, s17-18.

Dunkle, K. L., & Decker, M. R. (2013, Feb). Gender-based violence and HIV: reviewing the evidence for links and causal pathways in the general population and high-risk groups. *Am J Reprod Immunol, 69 Suppl 1*, 20-26. https://doi.org/10.1111/aji.12039

English, A. (Jan 1). Mandatory Reporting of Human Trafficking: Potential Benefits and Risks of Harm. *AMA J Ethics, 19*(1), 54-62.

English, A. (2017, Jan 1). Mandatory Reporting of Human Trafficking: Potential Benefits and Risks of Harm. *AMA J Ethics, 19*(1), 54-62. https://doi.org/10.1001/journalofethics.2017.19.1.pfor1-1701

Epidemic early syphilis--Montgomery County, Alabama, 1990-1991. (1992, Oct 23). *MMWR Morb Mortal Wkly Rep, 41*(42), 790-794.

Epstein, H. (2007). *The Invisible Cure*. Picador.

Essuon, A. D., Zhao, H., Wang, G., Collins, N., Karch, D., & Rao, S. (2020, Jan 31). HIV Testing Outcomes Among Blacks or African Americans - 50 Local U.S. Jurisdictions Accounting for the Majority of New HIV Diagnoses and Seven States with Disproportionate Occurrences of HIV in Rural Areas, 2017. *MMWR Morb Mortal Wkly Rep, 69*(4), 97-102. https://doi.org/10.15585/mmwr.mm6904a2

Ethical issues in the NIMH Collaborative HIV/STD Prevention Trial. (2007, Apr). *Aids, 21 Suppl 2*, S69-80. https://doi.org/10.1097/01.aids.0000266459.49138.b3

Ewuoso, C. (2019, May 26). Addressing the conflict between partner notification and patient confidentiality in serodiscordant relationships: How can Ubuntu help? *Dev World Bioeth*. https://doi.org/10.1111/dewb.12232

Fairchild, A. L., & Bayer, R. (2011, Aug 25). HIV surveillance, public health, and clinical medicine--will the walls come tumbling down? *N Engl J Med, 365*(8), 685-687. https://doi.org/10.1056/NEJMp1107294

Farmer, P. (1999). *Infection and Inequalities*. University of California Press.

Fischl, M. A., Richman, D. D., Grieco, M. H., Gottlieb, M. S., Volberding, P. A., Laskin, O. L., Leedom, J. M., Groopman, J. E., Mildvan, D., Schooley, R. T., & et al. (1987, Jul 23). The efficacy of azidothymidine (AZT) in the treatment of patients with AIDS and AIDS-related complex. A double-blind, placebo-controlled trial. *N Engl J Med, 317*(4), 185-191. https://doi.org/10.1056/nejm198707233170401

Forbes, K. M., Lomax, N., Cunningham, L., Hardie, J., Noble, H., Sarner, L., & Anderson, J. (2008, Jul). Partner notification in pregnant women with HIV: findings from three inner-city clinics. *HIV Med, 9*(6), 433-435. https://doi.org/10.1111/j.1468-1293.2008.00580.x

Gibbs, J., Sonnenberg, P., & Estcourt, C. S. (2017, Feb). Confidentiality of sexual health patients' information - what has history taught us and where do we stand? *Sex Transm Infect, 93*(1), 2. https://doi.org/10.1136/sextrans-2016-053002

Gielen, A. C., Fogarty, L., O'Campo, P., Anderson, J., Keller, J., & Faden, R. (2000, Sep). Women living with HIV: disclosure, violence, and social support. *J Urban Health, 77*(3), 480-491. https://doi.org/10.1007/bf02386755

Global HIV & AIDS statistics — 2019 fact sheet. (2019). https://www.unaids.org/en/resources/fact-sheet

Golub, S. A., & Indyk, D. (2006). HIV-infected individuals as partners in prevention: a redefinition of the partner notification process. *Soc Work Health Care, 42*(3-4), 225-235. https://doi.org/10.1300/J010v42n03_14

Gostin, L., & Curran, W. J. (1986, Dec). The limits of compulsion in controlling AIDS. *Hastings Cent Rep, 16*(6), suppl 24-29.

Gostin, L., & Curran, W. J. (1987, Feb). Legal control measures for AIDS: reporting requirements, surveillance, quarantine, and regulation of public meeting places. *Am J Public Health, 77*(2), 214-218. https://doi.org/10.2105/ajph.77.2.214

Grinsztejn, B., Hosseinipour, M. C., Ribaudo, H. J., Swindells, S., Eron, J., Chen, Y. Q., Wang, L., Ou, S. S., Anderson, M., McCauley, M., Gamble, T., Kumarasamy, N., Hakim, J. G., Kumwenda, J., Pilotto, J. H., Godbole, S. V., Chariyalertsak, S., de Melo, M. G., Mayer, K. H., Eshleman, S. H., Piwowar-Manning, E., Makhema, J., Mills, L. A., Panchia, R., Sanne, I., Gallant, J., Hoffman, I., Taha, T. E., Nielsen-Saines, K., Celentano, D., Essex, M., Havlir, D., & Cohen, M. S. (Apr). Effects of early versus delayed initiation of antiretroviral treatment on clinical outcomes of HIV-1 infection: results from the phase 3 HPTN 052 randomised controlled trial. *Lancet Infect Dis, 14*(4), 281-290.

Gruskin, S., & Tarantola, D. (2001). HIV/AIDS and human rights revisited. *Can HIV AIDS Policy Law Rev, 6*(1-2), 24-29.

Gunn, R. A., Montes, J. M., Toomey, K. E., Rolfs, R. T., Greenspan, J. R., Spitters, C. E., & Waterman, S. H. (1995, Jan-Feb). Syphilis in San Diego County 1983-1992: crack cocaine, prostitution, and the limitations of partner notification. *Sex Transm Dis, 22*(1), 60-66.

Guy, R., El-Hayek, C., Fairley, C. K., Wand, H., Carr, A., McNulty, A., Hoy, J., Bourne, C., McAllister, J., Tee, B. K., Baker, D., Roth, N., Stoove, M., & Chen, M. (2013). Opt-out and opt-in testing increases syphilis screening of HIV-positive men who have sex with men in Australia. *PLoS One, 8*(8), e71436. https://doi.org/10.1371/journal.pone.0071436

Hampton, T. (2008, Apr 23). Researchers seek ways to stem STDs: "alarming" STD rates found in teenaged girls. *Jama, 299*(16), 1888-1889. https://doi.org/10.1001/jama.299.16.1888

Health, I. D. o. P. (2015). *AIDS Confidentiality Act.* . https://www.dph.illinois.gov/topics-services2fdiseases-and-conditions2fhiv-aids%23laws-rules-laws-rules-hivaids

Hildesheimer, G. M. (2002). AIDS, partner notification and gender issues. *Med Law, 21*(1), 165-177.

HIV Prevention Act would require HIV reporting. (1997, May). *AIDS Alert, 12*(5), 54-55.

Ho, D. D. (1995, Aug 17). Time to hit HIV, early and hard. *N Engl J Med, 333*(7), 450-451. https://doi.org/10.1056/nejm199508173330710

Hyman, J. M., Li, J., & Stanley, E. A. (1999, Feb). The differential infectivity and staged progression models for the transmission of HIV. *Math Biosci, 155*(2), 77-109.

Is partner notification in the public interest? (1999, Oct). *Sex Transm Infect, 75*(5), 354-357. https://doi.org/10.1136/sti.75.5.354

James, J. S. (1996, Jul 19). Vancouver in perspective. *AIDS Treat News*(no 251), 1-3.

John, S. A., Walsh, J. L., Cho, Y. I., & Weinhardt, L. S. (2018, Feb). Perceived Risk of Intimate Partner Violence Among STI Clinic Patients: Implications for Partner Notification and Patient-Delivered Partner Therapy. *Arch Sex Behav, 47*(2), 481-492. https://doi.org/10.1007/s10508-017-1051-0

Kabengele Mpinga, E., Koya, M., Hasselgard-Rowe, J., Jeannot, E., Rehani, S. B., & Chastonay, P. (Dec). Rape in Armed Conflicts in the Democratic Republic of Congo: A Systematic Review of the Scientific Literature. *Trauma Violence Abuse, 18*(5), 581-592.

Kanny, D., Jeffries, W. L. t., Chapin-Bardales, J., Denning, P., Cha, S., Finlayson, T., & Wejnert, C. (Sep 20). Racial/Ethnic Disparities in HIV Preexposure Prophylaxis Among Men Who Have Sex with Men - 23 Urban Areas, 2017. *MMWR Morb Mortal Wkly Rep, 68*(37), 801-806.

Kerani, R. P., Handsfield, H. H., Stenger, M. S., Shafii, T., Zick, E., Brewer, D., & Golden, M. R. (2007, Mar). Rising rates of syphilis in the era of syphilis elimination. *Sex Transm Dis, 34*(3), 154-161. https://doi.org/10.1097/01.olq.0000233709.93891.e5

Ketels, B., & Vander Beken, T. (2012, Summer). Medical confidentiality and partner notification in cases of sexually transmissible infections in Belgium. *Med Law Rev, 20*(3), 399-422. https://doi.org/10.1093/medlaw/fws010

Kissinger, P. J., Niccolai, L. M., Magnus, M., Farley, T. A., Maher, J. E., Richardson-Alston, G., Dorst, D., Myers, L., & Peterman, T. A. (2003, Jan). Partner notification for HIV and syphilis: effects on sexual behaviors and relationship stability. *Sex Transm Dis, 30*(1), 75-82.

Koenig, L. J., & Moore, J. (2000, Jun). Women, violence, and HIV: a critical evaluation with implications for HIV services. *Matern Child Health J, 4*(2), 103-109.

Lamboi, S. E., & Sy, F. S. (1989, Winter). The impact of AIDS on state public health legislation in the United States: a critical review. *AIDS Educ Prev, 1*(4), 324-339.

Laurencin, C. T., Christensen, D. M., & Taylor, E. D. (2008, Jan). HIV/AIDS and the African-American community: a state of emergency. *J Natl Med Assoc, 100*(1), 35-43. https://doi.org/10.1016/s0027-9684(15)31172-x

Levine, M. L. (1988, Fall). Contact tracing for HIV infection: a plea for privacy. *Columbia Human Rights Law Rev, 20*(1), 157-201.

Lichtenstein, B. (2003, Dec). Stigma as a barrier to treatment of sexually transmitted infection in the American deep south: issues of race, gender and poverty. *Soc Sci Med, 57*(12), 2435-2445. https://doi.org/10.1016/j.socscimed.2003.08.002

Liu, B. C. C., & Vaughn, M. S. (May-Jun). Legal and policy issues from the United States and internationally about mandatory reporting of child abuse. *Int J Law Psychiatry, 64*, 219-229.

Lundgren, J. D., Babiker, A. G., Gordin, F., Emery, S., Grund, B., Sharma, S., Avihingsanon, A., Cooper, D. A., Fätkenheuer, G., Llibre, J. M., Molina, J. M., Munderi, P., Schechter, M., Wood, R., Klingman, K. L., Collins, S., Lane, H. C., Phillips, A. N., & Neaton, J. D. (2015, Aug 27). Initiation of Antiretroviral Therapy in Early Asymptomatic HIV Infection. *N Engl J Med, 373*(9), 795-807. https://doi.org/10.1056/NEJMoa1506816

Lunny, C., & Shearer, B. D. (2011, Dec). A systematic review and comparison of HIV contact tracing laws in Canada. *Health Policy, 103*(2-3), 111-123. https://doi.org/10.1016/j.healthpol.2011.07.011

Magadi, M. A. (2013, Jun). The disproportionate high risk of HIV infection among the urban poor in sub-Saharan Africa. *AIDS Behav, 17*(5), 1645-

1654. https://doi.org/10.1007/s10461-012-0217-y

Maher, J. E., Peterson, J., Hastings, K., Dahlberg, L. L., Seals, B., Shelley, G., & Kamb, M. L. (2000, Nov 1). Partner violence, partner notification, and women's decisions to have an HIV test. *J Acquir Immune Defic Syndr, 25*(3), 276-282.

Mayer, K. H., Sohn, A., Kippax, S., & Bras, M. (2018, Jul). Addressing HIV criminalization: science confronts ignorance and bias. *J Int AIDS Soc, 21*(7), e25163. https://doi.org/10.1002/jia2.25163

McDonald, E. A., Currie, M. J., & Bowden, F. J. (2006, Dec). Delayed diagnosis of HIV: missed opportunities and triggers for testing in the Australian Capital Territory. *Sex Health, 3*(4), 291-295.

Monroe-Wise, A., Maingi Mutiti, P., Kimani, H., Moraa, H., Bukusi, D. E., & Farquhar, C. (2019, Jul). Assisted partner notification services for patients receiving HIV care and treatment in an HIV clinic in Nairobi, Kenya: a qualitative assessment of barriers and opportunities for scale-up. *J Int AIDS Soc, 22 Suppl 3*, e25315. https://doi.org/10.1002/jia2.25315

Montoy, J. C., Dow, W. H., & Kaplan, B. C. (2016, Jan 19). Patient choice in opt-in, active choice, and opt-out HIV screening: randomized clinical trial. *Bmj, 532*, h6895. https://doi.org/10.1136/bmj.h6895

Myers, T., Worthington, C., Haubrich, D. J., Ryder, K., & Calzavara, L. (2003, Aug). HIV testing and counseling: test providers' experiences of best practices. *AIDS Educ Prev, 15*(4), 309-319.

New guidelines on HIV testing and partner notification. (1992, Dec 18). *Commun Dis Rep CDR Wkly, 2*(51), 231.

New York issues draft rules for notification, surveillance. (1999, Apr 2). *AIDS Policy Law, 14*(6), 1, 6-7.

Nie, J. B., Walker, S. T., Qiao, S., Li, X., & Tucker, J. D. (2015). Truth-telling to the patient, family, and the sexual partner: a rights approach to the role of healthcare providers in adult HIV disclosure in China. *AIDS Care, 27 Suppl 1*, 83-89. https://doi.org/10.1080/09540121.2015.1071772

O'Brien, R. C. (1993, Fall). The legal dilemma of partner notification during the HIV epidemic. *J Clin Ethics, 4*(3), 245-252.

Omunakwe, H. E., Okoye, H., Efobi, C., Onodingene, M., Chinenye, S., & Nwauche, C. A. (2015, Sep). Disclosure amongst adult HIV patients on antiretroviral therapy in Port Harcourt, Nigeria. *Int J STD AIDS, 26*(10), 729-732. https://doi.org/10.1177/0956462414552815

Onotai, L. O., Nwaorgu, O. G., & Okoye, B. C. (2004, Jul-Sep). Ethical issues in HIV/AIDS infections. *Niger J Med, 13*(3), 282-285.

Outbreak of primary and secondary syphilis--Baltimore City, Maryland, 1995. (1996, Mar 1). *MMWR Morb Mortal Wkly Rep, 45*(8), 166-169.

Park, J. (Dec). Historical Origins of the Tuskegee Experiment: The Dilemma of Public Health in the United States. *Uisahak, 26*(3), 545-578.

Parran, T. (1937). *Shadow on the Land. Syphilis. New York:* . Reynal & Hitchcock, .

Parran, T. (1938a, Mar). Concerning the conquest of syphilis and gonorrhea. A statement from Surgeon-General Thomas Parran. *Cal West Med, 48*(3), 215.

Parran, T. (1938b, Feb 18). SYPHILIS: A PUBLIC HEALTH PROBLEM. *Science, 87*(2251), 147-152. https://doi.org/10.1126/science.87.2251.147

Partner notification. (1998, Oct 30). *AIDS Policy Law, 13*(20), 16.

Partner notification for preventing HIV infection. (1991, Nov 2). *Lancet, 338*(8775), 1112-1113.

Partner notification for preventing human immunodeficiency virus (HIV) infection--Colorado, Idaho, South Carolina, Virginia. (1988, Jul 1). *MMWR Morb Mortal Wkly Rep, 37*(25), 393-396, 401-392.

Patterson, S. E., Milloy, M. J., Ogilvie, G., Greene, S., Nicholson, V., Vonn, M., Hogg, R., & Kaida, A. (2015). The impact of criminalization of HIV non-disclosure on the healthcare engagement of women living with HIV in Canada: a comprehensive review of the evidence. *J Int AIDS Soc, 18*(1), 20572. https://doi.org/10.7448/ias.18.1.20572

Peterman, T. A., Su, J., Bernstein, K. T., & Weinstock, H. (2015, Feb). Syphilis in the United States: on the rise? *Expert Rev Anti Infect Ther, 13*(2), 161-168. https://doi.org/10.1586/14787210.2015.990384

Plotzker, R. E., Murphy, R. D., & Stoltey, J. E. (2018, Sep). Congenital Syphilis Prevention: Strategies, Evidence, and Future Directions. *Sex Transm Dis, 45*(9S Suppl 1), S29-s37. https://doi.org/10.1097/olq.0000000000000846

Polansky, A., Levy, I., & Mor, Z. (2019, Sep). Risk factors of syphilis co-infection among HIV-infected men who have sex with men in Tel-Aviv, Israel. *AIDS Care, 31*(9), 1157-1161. https://doi.org/10.1080/09540121.2019.1612006

Primary and secondary syphilis - Jefferson county, Alabama, 2002-2007. (2009, May 8). *MMWR Morb Mortal Wkly Rep, 58*(17), 463-467.

Public Health Service guidelines for counseling and antibody testing to prevent HIV infection and AIDS. (1987, Aug 14). *MMWR Morb Mortal*

Wkly Rep, 36(31), 509-515.

Quinn, C., Nakyanjo, N., Ddaaki, W., Burke, V. M., Hutchinson, N., Kagaayi, J., Wawer, M. J., Nalugoda, F., & Kennedy, C. E. (2018, Oct). HIV Partner Notification Values and Preferences Among Sex Workers, Fishermen, and Mainland Community Members in Rakai, Uganda: A Qualitative Study. *AIDS Behav, 22*(10), 3407-3416. https://doi.org/10.1007/s10461-018-2035-3

Reif, S. S., Whetten, K., Wilson, E. R., McAllaster, C., Pence, B. W., Legrand, S., & Gong, W. (2014). HIV/AIDS in the Southern USA: a disproportionate epidemic. *AIDS Care, 26*(3), 351-359. https://doi.org/10.1080/09540121.2013.824535

Reverby, S. M. (May 14). Listening to narratives from the Tuskegee syphilis study. *Lancet, 377*(9778), 1646-1647.

Rodríguez, M. A., McLoughlin, E., Nah, G., & Campbell, J. C. (2001, Aug 1). Mandatory reporting of domestic violence injuries to the police: what do emergency department patients think? *Jama, 286*(5), 580-583. https://doi.org/10.1001/jama.286.5.580

Rose, J. W. (2001, Mar). To tell or not to tell. Legislative imposition of partner notification duties for HIV patients. *J Leg Med, 22*(1), 107-123. https://doi.org/10.1080/019476401750171179

Rosenfeld, E. A., Marx, J., Terry, M. A., Stall, R., Pallatino, C., Borrero, S., & Miller, E. (2016, Jul). Intimate partner violence, partner notification, and expedited partner therapy: a qualitative study. *Int J STD AIDS, 27*(8), 656-661. https://doi.org/10.1177/0956462415591938

Rothenberg, K. H., & Paskey, S. J. (1995, Nov). The risk of domestic violence and women with HIV infection: implications for partner notification, public policy, and the law. *Am J Public Health, 85*(11), 1569-1576. https://doi.org/10.2105/ajph.85.11.1569

Rubin, R. (Feb 26). Why Are Mothers Still Passing Syphilis to Their Babies? *Jama, 321*(8), 729-731.

Saag, M. S., Benson, C. A., Gandhi, R. T., Hoy, J. F., Landovitz, R. J., Mugavero, M. J., Sax, P. E., Smith, D. M., Thompson, M. A., Buchbinder, S. P., Del Rio, C., Eron, J. J., Jr., Fätkenheuer, G., Günthard, H. F., Molina, J. M., Jacobsen, D. M., & Volberding, P. A. (2018, Jul 24). Antiretroviral Drugs for Treatment and Prevention of HIV Infection in Adults: 2018 Recommendations of the International Antiviral Society-USA Panel. *Jama, 320*(4), 379-396. https://doi.org/10.1001/jama.2018.8431

Sovran, S. (2013, Mar). Understanding culture and HIV/AIDS in sub-Saharan Africa. *Sahara J, 10*(1), 32-41. https://doi.org/10.1080/17290376.2013.807071

Stone, V. E. (2012, Feb). HIV/AIDS in Women and Racial/Ethnic Minorities in the U.S. *Curr Infect Dis Rep, 14*(1), 53-60. https://doi.org/10.1007/s11908-011-0226-4

Tan, W. S., Chen, M., Ivan, M., Stone, K., Rane, V., Fairley, C. K., & Ong, J. J. (2016, Nov). Partner Notification Outcomes for Men Who Have Sex With Men Diagnosed With Syphilis Referred to Partner Notification Officers, Melbourne, Australia. *Sex Transm Dis, 43*(11), 685-689. https://doi.org/10.1097/olq.0000000000000512

Tesoriero, J. M., Battles, H. B., Heavner, K., Leung, S. Y., Nemeth, C., Pulver, W., & Birkhead, G. S. (2008, Apr). The effect of name-based reporting and partner notification on HIV testing in New York State. *Am J Public Health, 98*(4), 728-735. https://doi.org/10.2105/ajph.2007.092742

Thomas, D. R., Williams, C. J., Andrady, U., Anderson, V., Humphreys, S., Midgley, C. M., Fina, L., Craine, N., Porter-Jones, G., Wilde, A., & Whiteside, C. (2016, Aug). Outbreak of syphilis in men who have sex with men living in rural North Wales (UK) associated with the use of social media. *Sex Transm Infect, 92*(5), 359-364. https://doi.org/10.1136/sextrans-2015-052323

Using the Internet for partner notification of sexually transmitted diseases--Los Angeles County, California, 2003. (2004, Feb 20). *MMWR Morb Mortal Wkly Rep, 53*(6), 129-131.

Vancouver AIDS conference: special report. The epidemic now: current status and latest trends of HIV / AIDS in Africa -- a consensus update. (1996, Aug-Sep). *AIDS Anal Afr, 6*(4), 14-15.

Walcott, D. M., Cerundolo, P., & Beck, J. C. (2001). Current analysis of the Tarasoff duty: an evolution towards the limitation of the duty to protect. *Behav Sci Law, 19*(3), 325-343.

Walters, D. J. (1996, Sep 15). Powerful politics at the XI International Conference on AIDS. *Cmaj, 155*(6), 712-713.

Ward, J. W., Holmberg, S. D., Allen, J. R., Cohn, D. L., Critchley, S. E., Kleinman, S. H., Lenes, B. A., Ravenholt, O., Davis, J. R., Quinn, M. G., & et al. (1988, Feb 25). Transmission of human immunodeficiency virus (HIV) by blood transfusions screened as negative for HIV antibody. *N Engl J Med, 318*(8), 473-478. https://doi.org/10.1056/nejm198802253180803

WHO Guidelines Approved by the Guidelines Review Committee. (2016). In *Guidelines on HIV Self-Testing and Partner Notification: Supplement to Consolidated Guidelines on HIV Testing Services*. World Health Organization

WHO Guidelines Approved by the Guidelines Review Committee. Guidelines on HIV Self-Testing and Partner Notification: Supplement to Consolidated Guidelines on HIV Testing Services. Geneva: World Health Organization. (2016). who.int/hiv/pub/vct/hiv-self-testing-guidelines/eng/

Williams, I. G., & De Cock, K. M. (1996, Oct). The XI international conference on AIDS. Vancouver 7-12 July 1996. A review of Clinical Science Track B. *Genitourin Med, 72*(5), 365-369. https://doi.org/10.1136/sti.72.5.365

Chapter Three

Embedding HIV into the Undergraduate College Course

Shan-Estelle Brown, PhD
Department of Anthropology, Rollins College

Abstract

Undergraduate students represent an important population to address HIV because studies have shown that this population's knowledge of HIV prevention may be low. The generational group known as post-millennials was born after the worldwide dissemination of antiretroviral medications and may be complacent about HIV. Given that youth worldwide account for over 20% of new HIV infections and that some areas of the United States are currently experiencing increases in new diagnoses, the imperative is to provide education alongside advocating for structural change. I argue that to preserve the memory of HIV and honor the lives of people past and present with HIV, HIV information and narratives still need to be taught and should be embedded in curricula of different sizes with an emphasis on building empathy and empowerment. I use as an example my fifteen-week medical anthropology course, "Drugs, Sex, and HIV" which centers on the HIV pandemic with particular focus on the ways that inequality has made some populations more vulnerable to HIV than others. I also argue that we need more teaching professionals to become comfortable, competent, and adept at teaching topics like HIV to maintain a broad coalition of HIV-informed people.

Embedding HIV into the Undergraduate College Course

HIV is an important disease to study from a social science perspective because the HIV pandemic has a well-documented, recent history that highlights the existing vulnerabilities of every country on earth. HIV contains multitudes. HIV tells the story of problems of access to medical care, underfunded public health infrastructures, activism in the absence of political will, health inequality, narratives of survival, conspiracy theories, persisting stereotypes and entrenched stigma about HIV and people living with HIV. The discourse around HIV is changing and moving out of language of crisis and exceptionalism and further chronic disease. There is still no cure or vaccine for HIV, but the disease is preventable. We have numerous models to compare responses to HIV to know what works, but the number of cases is still high and growing in some places. In this essay, I argue that higher education needs to focus increased attention on teaching about HIV in a variety of disciplinary settings if we are to successfully inform the next generation of professionals entering the workforce who will encounter and need to have empathy for people living with HIV in their daily lives. First, I summarize the historical disciplinary locations for teaching HIV, anthropological approaches to HIV, youth perspectives on HIV, and finally I describe my semester-length course on HIV designed for an undergraduate audience at a small liberal arts college.

Which Disciplines Teach HIV?

I conducted a literature review on studies on HIV and undergraduates and found that the majority of studies pose students as the research subjects whose seroprevalance is tested and where they are surveyed for their HIV knowledge, attitudes, and behaviors, and much less often, how an undergraduate course affects HIV risk (Marsiglia et al., 2013). A glaring omission, however, is that there is little research for how or where these students actually acquired this knowledge, even if it can be difficult to understand how students apply the knowledge they might have attained. Courses specifically addressing HIV at the undergraduate level are scarce, as the majority of literature on teaching HIV is directed at undergraduate nursing and medical students, not 4-year undergraduate college students. We can identify where learning about HIV is not happening. One study tried to work backwards to understand HIV knowledge at the undergraduate level by assessing medical and dental school students (Carter, Greenfield, & Kenkre, 1997). I reviewed articles on pedagogy about HIV and found that the following disciplines are the most common, listed in alphabetical order: Anthropology, Bioethics, Business/ Human Resources, Global/Public Health, History of Medicine, Psychology, Sociology, and Visual Arts. Across these disciplines, it seems to be a class here and there that ends up being written about for publication. A few business schools began in the mid 1990s teaching students about HIV to ensure that business students would be prepared to deal with HIV in the workplace (Kohl, Miller, & Miller, 1997; Miller, 2000, 2008; Miller, Backer, & Rogers, 1997). The majority of articles on HIV and pedagogy come from Sociology, probably out of a desire to address the relationships between this disease and society. Sociologists teaching HIV argued for embedding HIV into sociological courses by connecting HIV to sociological concepts such as the sociological imagination (Lichtenstein, 2010), cognitive dissonance, deviance, social problems, stratification, and social change (Brabant, 1991).

Undergraduate courses on HIV that have been published have used a variety of techniques such as using participatory visual methodologies to encourage collaboration across institutions (Tanga, de Lange, & van Laren, 2014), using problem-based learning (Eglitis, Buntman, & Alexander, 2016), encouraging students to participate in research as a way of doing anthropology (Copeland, 2016), and incorporating service learning to educate students about local HIV issues (Jones & Abes, 2003; Lena, 1995; Marullo, 1998). Of the authors who published articles about teaching HIV, the considerations are about viewing curriculum as enabling a complex conversation (De Lange, 2014), classroom management (Lichtenstein, 2010) and teaching topics deemed sensitive, including death (Caswell, 2010), race, sexual behavior, sexual orientation, and drug use (Lichtenstein, 2010; Lichtenstein & DeCoster, 2014; Lowe & Jones, 2010). The teaching environment itself has also been questioned, as one author described a "hostile environment" of teaching undergraduates in sociology in Louisiana (Brabant, 1991). Authors have also questioned the language about HIV in textbooks for psychology (Wong, Harper, Duffy, Faulring, & Eggleston, 2001) and sociology (Hunt, 1990; Weitz, 1992). Teaching HIV does mean a commitment to addressing challenges of teaching LGBT health care (Davy, Amsler, & Duncombe, 2015; Lim, Johnson, & Eliason, 2015). A particular concern raised is that discussing LGBT health care runs the risk of reinforcing health problems of MSM as products of their sexuality, in addition to more generalized issues of homophobia and transphobia (Davy et al., 2015). Despite the high numbers of women worldwide affected by HIV, there is not much information on undergraduate courses focusing even as a module specifically about HIV and women (Champeau & Shaw, 2003). Gay men and HIV remain inextricably linked to each other, and women's HIV issues remain underrepresented.

Curiosity and fear surrounding HIV have not changed much in US mainstream society because of durable norms. Students are still bringing into the classroom the snippets that they have heard; they know HIV as a "gay disease" even if infections in their own communities come primarily from heterosexual sex between partners whose HIV status is unknown. Rose Weitz (1989) identified the following issues of teaching undergraduate students about HIV: students taking her course because they are emotionally close to the topic; striking a balance between religious objections to homosexuality and protecting homosexual students in the course from harm; students' lack of knowledge about HIV (Weitz, 1989). The idea of protecting homosexual students from harm is echoed in this quote from Brabant (1991), the instructor who acknowledged working in the environment hostile to HIV, regarding students disclosing their HIV-positive status: "There is a tendency to want to tell someone or even everyone. Thus, it is important to prepare the HIV/AIDS affected student for re-entry into the environment from which he/she came. The student will return to the same conditions which forced secrecy in the first place. Discuss this fact with the student and suggest that it might be best not to confide in anyone else for at least a week" (Brabant, 1991, p. 492). Brabant is acknowledging that she has created an environment for students safe enough to disclose their HIV status in class, but the reality is that her students are not safe outside of class. Course goals in the early 1990s to demythologize and humanize HIV in undergraduate classrooms (Hunt, 1990; Klein, 1993) remain vitally important to the understanding of HIV; only the students in the seats have changed. Nearly twenty years after those early HIV courses, one author used HIV knowledge in his course to specifically to make a concerted effort to replace students' "catastrophic contagion" identified at the start of the course with encouragement and empowerment (Moremen, 2010). Certainly the humanity of people living with HIV should not be in doubt, yet it seems to be something to be argued and compared to the HIV "monsters" (Persson & Newman, 2008) deliberately constructed and perpetuated in mainstream media.

Anthropological Approaches to HIV

Today, there are hundreds of ethnographic books and articles on HIV written by anthropologists and other social scientists. Contrary to this prolific writing, anthropologists were initially slow to contribute to HIV research (Parker, 2001) and therefore, early epidemiological research on HIV lacked attention to broader social and cultural factors. According to Parker (2001), anthropologists began shifting HIV research from individualistic concerns to the investigation of cultural meanings, researching the impact of culture on behavior relating to HIV and drug use. Some of this work could be considered *témoignage* (Redfield, 2006), or the need to be a witness or speak out against inhumane injustices. Anthropologists have provided useful information in the study of drug use by gaining access to social settings where drugs are acquired and consumed. Direct observation of drug-related behaviors and risk activities happen has contributed to our understanding of HIV and Hepatitis C transmission through shared needles and understandings about motivations and drivers of sharing needles in the first place. Two camps developed, consisting of the "traditional" anthropologists who offered socio-cultural depth to biomedical and epidemiological understandings of the HIV/AIDS epidemic, and the critical medical anthropologists who advocated for changing unequal societal structures, using structural violence as the principal perspective for understanding HIV/AIDS (Baer, Singer, & Susser, 1997). By distinguishing vulnerability from risk, the CMA anthropologists uncovered the mechanisms that made individuals and communities at increased risk for HIV. I spoke to some anthropologists through our listserv on AIDS and Anthropology, and respondents stated that in their courses, they tend to assign an ethnography with articles, but very few are teaching HIV as a full semester course. One other anthropologist, like me, used HIV as a frame for a deeper understanding of understanding poverty and power. Looking at introductory medical anthropology course syllabi, I identify that most courses spend a week of course material and attention specifically to HIV.

Teaching Millennials and Gen Z about HIV

Over thirty years of teaching undergraduates about HIV, courses seem to have been tailored to the academic and broader social environments in which they are situated. Although it appears that the focus heretofore has not traditionally been on the "audience" or recipients of HIV information in an undergraduate classroom, I am arguing that any module or course on HIV going forward should convey relevance to students and incorporate technology and social media because they are digital natives. Millennials (Generation Y, born 1981-1996) and Generation Z (born 1997 and onward, according to Pew Research Center (Dimock, 2019)) are known to be highly tech savvy and interested in questioning and changing the status quo (Jiang & Anderson, 2018), but despite having much information at their fingertips, their knowledge base tends to be shallow. Gen Z students still need critical thinking, information literacy, and increased empathy for other humans. For students born after 1996, teaching HIV is teaching them the recent history before their births; these students were born after the peak of HIV deaths, and they have enough awareness of medication to minimize HIV to just another treatable chronic disease without really knowing the twists and turns in getting to this point.

While some students may have benefited from age-appropriate instruction about HIV as elementary school students like that described by Walsh and Bibace (1990), gaps in their knowledge about HIV may come from silence about sex, class and race and the infiltration of abstinence-only education into their schools, so that by the time they get to college, they have inherited stigma about HIV passed down from previous generations and received a variety of mixed messages about sex and infectious disease. Having been born after the advent of antiretroviral medications, their messages about HIV may have begun in grade school and framed reductively as chronic disease. This sentiment is reflected by Salhi and Brown (2019) who provide an explanation for why their students seem disinterested in HIV compared to other human rights topics they presented: "we believe that it was the very *success* of health and human rights activism that made the suffering associated with HIV/AIDS seem like a historical relic or a lackluster example for most of our students" (199). There is a persistent question of HIV exceptionalism (Benton, 2012, 2015; Moyer & Hardon, 2014; Smith, Ahmed, & Whiteside, 2011), the belief that HIV should be addressed and funded as a disease different from other infectious diseases or even other sexually transmitted infections, which may question the future utility of teaching about HIV independently of infectious disease or other STIs or teaching a full course on HIV. As HIV discourses continue to move out of a language and tone of crisis and into long-term care and medical home models that treat HIV as one more disease in their care, it is possible that the further downplaying of HIV may be an indicator of increasingly successful disease control. Until HIV is cured, or a vaccine discovered, or the numbers of new diagnoses becomes remarkably small, it would seem that a course on HIV could be relegated solely to history.

The new challenge is to increase HIV knowledge for these age groups. A 2019 study by Merck and Prevention Access Campaign found that "23 percent of HIV-negative millennials — and 41 percent of HIV-negative Gen Z respondents — admitted they were either "not at all" informed or "only somewhat" informed about HIV. Nearly half of the HIV-negative respondents, who were all 18 to 36, said they believed the virus could be transmitted by someone whose viral load was undetectable," which is incorrect

(Avery, 2019). According to the World Health Organization, over 30% of all new HIV infections globally are estimated to occur among youth ages 15 to 25 years ("HIV and youth," 2020). According to the CDC, 21% of the new HIV diagnoses in the US and dependent areas in 2018 were among youth aged 13-24 ("HIV and youth," 2020). These statistics become vitally important for understanding HIV in the state where I teach.

HIV in Florida

Florida is a state with rising numbers of new HIV diagnoses during a time when most states are on the decline. Florida is a state of focus for the CDC's new campaign to end the HIV epidemic in the US (Centers for Disease Control and Prevention and Health Resources & Services Administration, 2020), and it is geographically part of a chain of southern states where the following issues confound the improvement of health outcomes: poverty, institutionalized and interpersonal stigma against PLWH and against LGBT and same-gender-loving people, institutionalized racism, and bans against needle and syringe exchange. Florida has not yet expanded Medicaid into the state, and in 2017, the state ranked 40th in public health funding as measured by spending from state and federal sources (Tobin, 2017). Sexually transmitted diseases are on the rise in the state, with none on the decline, and 119,000 people are living with HIV as of 2018, according to the Florida Department of Health (Florida Department of Health, 2019c). In the state, the highest proportion of persons who received an HIV diagnosis in Florida in 2018 were age 20–29; the two top populations receiving HIV diagnoses are men who have sex with men and female heterosexual women (Florida Department of Health, 2019c). Among Floridian men, MSM comprise 74% of the men who received an HIV diagnosis with Hispanic/Latino and Black men representing 37% and 35% of the 87,285 men in Florida living with HIV, respectively (Florida Department of Health, 2019b) Among Floridian women, Black women comprise 18% of all the HIV diagnoses and for them, the epidemic is driven overwhelmingly by heterosexual contact (96%) (Florida Department of Health, 2019a). In Florida public schools, each school district chooses between abstinence-only, abstinence-plus or comprehensive sexual health education instruction (Florida Department of Education, 2020). While not all students enrolling at my institution are from Florida, students come to college with a variety of gender and sexual stereotypes and varying sexual health knowledge, which becomes critical during and after adolescents' sexual debut, which varies by age and ethnicity in the United States (Cavazos-Rehg et al., 2009). Although sexual education is not specifically one of my course objectives, "setting the record straight" on how a person can and cannot get HIV is one of the first lessons.

Inspiration for My Course, "Drugs, Sex, and HIV"

My course, "Drugs, Sex, and HIV" is an attempt to narrate an intersectional, international story of HIV directed at millennials and Gen Zers to show them the intersections of culture, poverty, and disease and expand medical anthropology and global health offerings for my department. The course is a way for me to honor my five-year postdoctoral fellowship at Yale School of Medicine in the AIDS Program working on an interdisciplinary team. It is a different thing for graduate-level researchers to "talk shop" to each other compared to undergraduates with varying levels of HIV or anthropology knowledge. Thus, in this 300-level course, one can find Anthropology majors and minors, students aiming to fulfill a global health elective, and students simply interested in learning more about drugs, sex, or HIV. My overarching goal is for students to come away from the course with increased empathy for people living with HIV today, some historical and socio-cultural context for how the HIV pandemic unfolded, and recognition of the structural reasons that explain why we still see new diagnoses today. Since Spring 2017, I have taught the course four times. The variety of students and their interest in my course is interestingly no different from what Rose Weitz saw in her HIV course in 1989 (Weitz, 1989). For some students who finish the course, the course solidifies their interest in becoming health professionals; some students pursue graduate education such as master of public health, medical or veterinary school. Others become activated to directly fight HIV locally through service or international internships; one student used his HIV knowledge gained in the course to leverage a community engagement experience with a local HIV organization into a volunteer and then paid position. Other students have incorporated it into their research; two students from last year's class are now Fulbright Fellowship and Truman Scholarship recipients for HIV-focused research.

My goals for the course were designed using Bloom's taxonomy and are intended for anyone with little to no knowledge about HIV:

1) Understand how anthropologists approach and study the HIV pandemic.
2) Investigate the lived experiences of people living with or affected by HIV today.
3) Examine how the social determinants of health affect individuals with respect to substance use, sexual behavior, and HIV.

4) Evaluate future directions in HIV research, treatment, and prevention.
5) Become familiar with a range of current resources, including publications, (journals, books, data sources, ethnographies, films, etc.), online sources, professional associations and organizations, through which students can continue to learn about and contribute to the study of HIV.

Course Content

Discussing HIV is an opportunity to discuss the social determinants of health, health equity. The topics raised have direct connections to the United Nations Sustainable Development Goals. In the syllabus, a section called "Why should you want to study HIV?" is an attempt to draw students into the course:

HIV is a preventable disease caused by a virus. That's the short version of the story. Human Immunodeficiency Virus is also a pandemic, a worldwide spread of a new disease, that continues to be a major public and global health issue. Studying this pandemic will help us plan better for the next one. HIV is no longer a "death sentence," and in this class you'll learn why. You'll also learn how fear and stigma were and still are strong motivators in shaping human behavior and health policy. By understanding HIV, you understand humanity. If you are planning to work in a health career in the US or abroad, you will be equipped with the most up-to-date information to understand the intersections between human behavior, culture, and infectious disease.

The course is organized over the sixteen-week semester in two main halves; the first half is designed to present new information in modular form with a new module every 1-2 weeks. The topics are on the epidemiology of HIV, history of the pandemic with an emphasis on activism, medical discoveries, and missed political opportunities, HIV criminalization, anthropological approaches to the pandemic, risk and prevention as constructed categories, novel uses of social media, and stigma and access to care in the US South, especially among MSM. The second half turns to deeper investigation into the key populations affected by HIV today, starting with women, transgender people, incarcerated people, and how one's occupation can affect HIV risk. That week is a discussion about migrant workers such as miners, fishermen, and farmworkers, as well as sex workers. The course's second half risks being interpreted as repetitive because the main topics have already been introduced, but the focus on specific populations reinforces the ideas by providing deeper context into the ways that poverty, class, race, law, and gender intersect in communities around the world, provoking specific responses to achieve health equity. The second half of the course also shifts to the student conducting secondary research using country level-data from UNAIDS country reports and other sources to investigate HIV in-depth in a country of their choice to identify gaps in the report and opportunities for conducting original research to contributing to filling those gaps.

Course readings have a global focus and include articles by social scientists with an emphasis on articles by anthropologists and includes medical researchers, and reports from organizations like WHO, CDC, and UNAIDS. Despite ethnography being the main product of anthropologists, I do not assign whole ethnographies in this course because they are too lengthy for the module-based course format; also, not all students are versed in anthropology, and since it can take some time and page-length for anthropologists to tell important narratives about HIV, I use excerpts and research articles instead. Pictures really are worth thousands of words, and documentary films are extremely useful for storytelling about HIV and for conveying people's humanity and dignity during sickness. Not adhering to a textbook gives me the agility to curate readings to students' interests and as new HIV knowledge becomes available. When I first taught the course in 2017, PrEP was starting to gain increased public exposure despite being first approved by the US Food and Drug Administration in 2012. In the first iteration of the course, introducing PrEP happened at the end of the course as a "new frontier" and in a few short years, I have moved it to the second week of the course to make sure it is a part of what everyone should know about HIV. There is something satisfying in knowing that there has been some perceptible movement in HIV prevention.

Assignments begin with reading responses both structured from prompts and more open reactions from students. Three take home tests encourage students to apply what they have learned in class to a reading or film that they have not previously seen, or think in creative ways to develop an agenda for a health committee, a health poster or museum exhibit. Students give current events presentations on news articles of their choosing, so that I am not the only person making decisions about what we read and discuss. The culmination of the course involves a research project based on secondary research of a single country and a model-United Nations-style summit where students represent the countries they researched. This week-long event becomes important because students shift from describing what "they do" in a country to what "we do" and they collaborate in committees to develop resolutions.

What Students Say about the Course

I performed a content analysis of students' anonymous course evaluations. Students connect much of their enjoyment of the course to a professor's performance, and after disregarding comments relating to the professor, the following three themes emerged relating to the course itself: 1) the course's ability to increase students' knowledge about HIV's social factors; 2) the course's applicability to the world or understanding global complexities, and 3) the course's applicability to their own lives. Below are representative quotes from anonymous course feedback; each represents a different person.

The course's ability to increase students' knowledge about HIV's social factors:

> "The information was entirely new to me and the issues were never black-and-white. You really had to look at the issues with a sense of empathy while maintaining sensibility, because HIV's problems revolve entirely around socially mediated factors." (Spring 2017)

> "I am personally not interested in the course subject, but I gained knowledge and worked very hard in this class." (Spring 2017)

> "All of the topics discussed during this course was very interesting and all of the information was new to me which made this course very informational." (Fall 2017)

> "I feel like an HIV expert." (Fall 2017)

> "I learned so much more than I thought I would about HIV and all the social factors to it." (Spring 2019)

The course's applicability to the world or understanding global complexities:

> "It's so much more applicable to what I've been studying than I expected." (Spring 2017)

> "This class was amazing to learn about the diverse issues associated with the HIV/AIDS epidemic. I also learned a lot more about anthropology at the same time." (Spring 2019)

"I really did learn a lot more not just about what is going on in the US but all over the world." (Spring 2019)

The course's applicability to their own lives:

"I often find myself paying more attention to HIV/AIDS as a whole realizing the [e]ffects are still current in today's society." (Fall 2017)

"Thanks to this class, my knowledge on the epidemic has expanded to a point that the other day, I was able to sustain a complex conversation on the matter with a professional linked to the United Nations. I'm eager to learn and help more." (Spring 2019)

"I loved how applicable to the world this class was. We engaged in relevant topics that matter. We had to be creative in our writing responses along with some assignments. We got to work on things that mattered to our interests." (Spring 2020)

Each course has some meaningful milestones. The first milestone involves watching them adopt the epidemiological language in the first few weeks in order to understand global and local statistics on HIV. Next, students at some point in the semester engage in spontaneous comparisons of the kind of sexual education they received, and how; this introspection is useful because it is not led by me and shows them the diversity in information retained and messaging that a group of people enrolled in the same class could receive over their lifetimes. Students start to read about the structural inequalities that make people vulnerable to HIV, stigma and HIV criminalization against people living with HIV, and the multiple, structural reasons why viral suppression can be so difficult to achieve. Back-to-back, they watch "How to Survive a Plague" and feel inspired by the creativity of Act Up until they watch "Fire in the Blood" and become enraged at pharmaceutical companies and governments blocking access to low-cost antiretroviral medications. Students who have some familiarity with HIV might enter the course with a patronizing tone about HIV infection in that new infections result from a lack of education and later finish the course advocating for the adoption of needle and syringe exchange in their home communities.

Put Meaningful Discussions of HIV Everywhere

Discussing HIV has the potential to change minds and remove stereotypes about drug users, sex workers, and all the other people without conveniently named categories who can get HIV. Students need time to understand the epidemiological terminology, such as viral suppression and how to use some of the language that categorizes people, such as "people living with HIV" or "men who have sex with men" compared to "gay men." The students I encounter are students who have "opted in" to learn about HIV, and so some potentially difficult discussions do not happen, such as arguments between students about deservingness and whether or not someone "deserved HIV" based on a transgression.

We can capitalize on Gen Zers' desire to lead meaningful lives by showing them what has already been lost and accomplished regarding the HIV pandemic and what still needs to be done. Incorporating discussions about HIV into undergraduate classroom settings are important, and certainly do not need to be done over a full semester. An important consideration is the need to help students discern between information, misinformation, and disinformation that they come across on the Internet or on social media. Social media also has the ability to point to reputable news sources and narratives of people living in joy. A music course can instruct students about activist musicians, lyrics about HIV, or the use of music concerts for gathering people together for HIV testing. An art class can present the work of artists affected by HIV, activist posters, and encourage students to deconstruct medical marketing advertisements. A political science or human rights course can address the indifference of the Reagan era, policies of forced sterilizations of women with HIV, HIV criminalization and laws against homosexuality and sex work. We need more teaching professionals to become comfortable, competent, and adept at teaching topics like HIV to maintain a broad coalition of HIV-informed people. These professionals need to feel empowered and equipped to teach "sensitive topics" related to the HIV pandemic at age-appropriate and knowledge-appropriate levels. Collaborations with local non-government organizations can produce meaningful service-learning experiences; collaborations with archives can provide students with the depth and historical context that they might lack. All of this teaching could benefit from trauma-informed pedagogy (Carello & Butler, 2015) to prevent traumatizing or re-traumatizing students.

On Teaching Pandemics during Pandemics

My personal experience of the first part of 2020 has been a strange one, as the semester involved teaching this course and Introduction to Public Health, a core course for the Global Health minor, and a course I teach every semester. In that course, I discuss pandemics and municipal planning in the context of influenza, particularly the 1918 influenza pandemic. Students write their first graded essay playing a pandemic-simulation game where they modify a pathogen to increase its infectious potential and compare global responses seen in the game to real-world public health responses. No matter where I turned, the in-class discussion was about pandemics, and then in mid-March my college abruptly transitioned, as so many institutions did, from in-person to virtual synchronous instruction. The students in both courses had to adjust; among numerous worries, I was concerned that the students in the HIV class would not want to discuss COVID-19. Instead, at their insistence, we had numerous discussions about COVID-19 based on what they were seeing from news around the world and in their home communities and drew parallels between HIV and COVID-19. We discussed whether or not comparisons between the two pandemics were warranted, which inspired a take-home exam question.

The Way Forward

Over the next few years we will see a proliferation of courses on the COVID-19 pandemic at the undergraduate and graduate levels, as this pandemic has swiftly changed all our lives. Other pandemics remain, and people are dealing with HIV and COVID-19 simultaneously, which will continue to exhaust the limited public health resources that we already have, as a result of decades of defunding that has rendered everyone vulnerable, but not equally. I also worry about "compassion fatigue" and the difficulty of students being able to revisit traumatic topics, and if the COVID-19 pandemic persists into the next year, some students may be intrigued to learn more about the environment they're living in, while others may reject the permeation of COVID-19 into their courses and treat it as further intrusion into their changed lives. The staying power of the COVID-19 courses will depend on being able to convey the relevance of studying pandemics and applying lessons learned from past pandemics to this one.

References

Avery, D. (2019). HIV from a hug? Misinformation persists among young Americans, study finds. Retrieved March 16, 2020, from https://www.nbcnews.com/feature/nbc-out/hiv-hug-misinformation-persists-among-young-americans-study-finds-n1090556

Baer, H. A., Singer, M., & Susser, I. (1997). *Medical anthropology and the world system: a critical perspective*. Westport, Conn. ; London: Bergin & Garvey.

Benton, A. (2012). Exceptional Suffering? Enumeration and Vernacular Accounting in the HIV-Positive Experience. *Medical Anthropology*, 31(4), 310-328. doi: 10.1080/01459740.2011.631959

Benton, A. (2015). *HIV exceptionalism: development through disease in Sierra Leone*. Minneapolis: University of Minnesota Press.

Brabant, S. (1991). Teaching about HIV Infection and AIDS in a Hostile Environment. *Teaching Sociology*, 19(4), 489-494. doi: 10.2307/1317892

Carello, J., & Butler, L. D. (2015). Practicing What We Teach: Trauma-Informed Educational Practice. *Journal of Teaching in Social Work*, 35(3), 262-278. doi: 10.1080/08841233.2015.1030059

Carter, Y. H., Greenfield, S. M., & Kenkre, J. E. (1997). A national survey to medical and dental schools to assess the level of undergraduate teaching and research about HIV/AIDS in the UK. Int J STD AIDS, 8(2), 88-94. doi: 10.1258/0956462971919624

Caswell, G. (2010). Teaching death studies: reflections from the classroom. *Enhancing Learning in the Social Sciences*, 2(3), 1-11. doi: 10.11120/elss.2010.02030009

Cavazos-Rehg, P. A., Krauss, M. J., Spitznagel, E. L., Schootman, M., Bucholz, K. K., Peipert, J. F., . . . Bierut, L. J. (2009). Age of sexual debut among US adolescents. *Contraception*, 80(2), 158-162. doi: 10.1016/j.contraception.2009.02.014

Centers for Disease Control and Prevention and Health Resources & Services Administration. (2020). Ending the HIV Epidemic Planning Program Guidance. Atlanta, GA: Centers for Disease Control and Prevention and Health Resources & Services Administration.

Champeau, D. A., & Shaw, S. M. (2003). Teaching about Interlocking Oppressions: The Case of HIV and Women. *Feminist Teacher*, 14(3), 208-219.

Copeland, T. (2016). Teaching the research process through student engagement: Cultural consensus analysis of HIV/AIDS. *Annals of*

Anthropological Practice, 40(2), 148-163. doi: 10.1111/napa.12098

Davy, Z., Amsler, S., & Duncombe, K. (2015). Facilitating LGBT Medical, Health and Social Care Content in Higher Education Teaching. *Qualitative Research in Education*, 4(2), 134-163.

De Lange, N. (2014). The HIV and AIDS academic curriculum in higher education. *South African Journal of Higher Education*, 28(2), 368-385.

Dimock, M. (2019). Defining generations: Where Millennials end and Generation Z begins. Retrieved September 17, 2019, from https://www.pewresearch.org/fact-tank/2019/01/17/where-millennials-end-and-generation-z-begins/

Eglitis, D. S., Buntman, F. L., & Alexander, D. V. (2016). Social Issues and Problem-based Learning in Sociology:Opportunities and Challenges in the Undergraduate Classroom. *Teaching Sociology*, 44(3), 212-220. doi: 10.1177/0092055x16643572

Florida Department of Education. (2020). Statutes, Policies & Guidelines. Retrieved May 20, 2020, from http://www.fldoe.org/schools/healthy-schools/sexual-edu/policies.stml

Florida Department of Health. (2019a). Black Women Living with an HIV Diagnosis in Florida, 2018: Florida Department of Health.

Florida Department of Health. (2019b). Men Living with an HIV Diagnosis in Florida, 2018: Florida Department of Health.

Florida Department of Health. (2019c). Persons Living with an HIV Diagnosis in Florida, 2018: Florida Department of Health.

HIV and youth. (2020). Retrieved May 23, 2020, from https://www.who.int/maternal_child_adolescent/topics/adolescence/hiv/en/

Hunt, C. W. (1990). Teaching Medical Sociology and AIDS: Some Ideas and Objectives. *Teaching Sociology*, 18(3), 303-312. doi: 10.2307/1317732

Jiang, J., & Anderson, M. (2018). Teens, Social Media & Technology 2018: Pew Research Center.

Jones, S. R., & Abes, E. S. (2003). Developing Student Understanding of HIV/AIDS through Community Service-Learning: A Case Study Analysis. *Journal of College Student Development*, 44(4), 470. doi: 10.1353/csd.2003.0040

Klein, H. (1993). Teaching a College-Level "AIDS and Society" Course. *Teaching Sociology*, 21(1), 1-12. doi: 10.2307/1318846

Kohl, J. P., Miller, A. N., & Miller, A. N. (1997). AIDS in the Workplace: The Response of American Business Schools. *Journal of Education for Business*, 73(2), 98-101. doi: 10.1080/08832329709601624

Lena, H. F. (1995). How Can Sociology Contribute to Integrating Service

Learning into Academic Curricula? *American Sociologist*, 26(4), 107. doi: 10.1007/BF02692359

Lichtenstein, B. (2010). Sensitive issues in the classroom: teaching about HIV in the American Deep South. *Enhancing Learning in the Social Sciences*, 2(3), 1-23. doi: 10.11120/elss.2010.02030002

Lichtenstein, B., & DeCoster, J. (2014). Lessons on Stigma:Teaching about HIV/AIDS. *Teaching Sociology*, 42(2), 140-150. doi: 10.1177/0092055x13510412

Lim, F., Johnson, M., & Eliason, M. (2015). A National Survey of Faculty Knowledge, Experience, and Readiness for Teaching Lesbian, Gay, Bisexual, and Transgender Health in Baccalaureate Nursing Programs. *Nursing Education Perspectives*, 36(3), 144-152. doi: 10.5480/14-1355

Lowe, P., & Jones, H. (2010). Teaching and Learning Sensitive Topics. *Enhancing Learning in the Social Sciences*, 2(3), 1-7. doi: 10.11120/elss.2010.02030001

Marsiglia, F. F., Jacobs, B. L., Nieri, T., Smith, S. J., Salamone, D., & Booth, J. (2013). Effects of an Undergraduate HIV/AIDS Course on Students' HIV Risk. *Journal of HIV/AIDS & Social Services*, 12(2), 172-189. doi: 10.1080/15381501.2013.790750

Marullo, S. (1998). Bringing Home Diversity: A Service-Learning Approach to Teaching Race and Ethnic Relations. *Teaching Sociology*, 26(4), 259-275. doi: 10.2307/1318767

Miller, A. N. (2000). Preparing Future Managers to Deal With AIDS/HIV in the Workplace. *Journal of Education for Business*, 75(5), 258. doi: 10.1080/08832320009599024

Miller, A. N. (2008). Teaching Business Students About HIV and AIDS in the Workplace: Curriculum and Resources. *Journal of Management Education*, 32(2), 210-227. doi: 10.1177/1052562907299721

Miller, A. N., Backer, T. E., & Rogers, E. M. (1997). Business education and the AIDS epidemic: Responding in the workplace. *Business Horizons*, 40(4), 78-86. doi: https://doi.org/10.1016/S0007-6813(97)90043-4

Moremen, R. D. (2010). One Starfish at a Time: Using Fundamentals in Sociology to Rethink Impressions about People Living with HIV/AIDS. *Teaching Sociology*, 38(2), 144-155.

Moyer, E., & Hardon, A. (2014). A Disease Unlike Any Other? Why HIV Remains Exceptional in the Age of Treatment. *Medical Anthropology*, 33(4), 263-269. doi: 10.1080/01459740.2014.890618

Parker, R. (2001). Sexuality, Culture, and Power in HIV/AIDS Research. *Annual Review of Anthropology*, 30(1), 163.

Persson, A., & Newman, C. (2008). Making monsters: heterosexuality, crime and race in recent Western media coverage of HIV. *Sociology of Health & Illness*, 30(4), 632-646. doi: doi:10.1111/j.1467-9566.2008.01082.x

Redfield, P. (2006). A Less Modest Witness: Collective Advocacy and Motivated Truth in a Medical Humanitarian Movement. *American Ethnologist*, 33(1), 3-26.

Salhi, B. A., & Brown, P. J. (2019). Teaching Health as a Human Right in the Undergraduate Context: Challenges and Opportunities. *Health and human rights*, 21(1), 191-202.

Smith, J., Ahmed, K., & Whiteside, A. (2011). Why HIV/AIDS should be treated as exceptional: arguments from sub-Saharan Africa and Eastern Europe. *African Journal of AIDS Research (AJAR)*, 10, 345-356. doi: 10.2989/16085906.2011.637736

Tanga, P., de Lange, N., & van Laren, L. (2014). 'Listening with our eyes': Collaboration and HIV and AIDS curriculum integration in South African higher education. *2014*, 10(1). doi: 10.4102/td.v10i1.18

Tobin, T. C. (2017, Dec 12, 2017). How is Florida's health? Not so great, report says. *Tampa Bay Times*. Retrieved from https://www.tampabay.com/news/health/How-is-Florida-s-health-Not-so-great-report-says_163533020/

Walsh, M. E., & Bibace, R. (1990). Developmentally-based AIDS/HIV education. *Journal of School Health*, 60, 256+.

Weitz, R. (1989). Confronting the Epidemic: Teaching about AIDS. *Teaching Sociology*, 17(3), 360-364. doi: 10.2307/1318086

Weitz, R. (1992). The Presentation of AIDS/HIV Disease in Introductory Sociology Textbooks. *Teaching Sociology*, 20(3), 239-243. doi: 10.2307/1319066

Wong, F. Y., Harper, G. W., Duffy, K. G., Faulring, C., & Eggleston, B. (2001). A content analysis of hiv/aids information in psychology textbooks: implications for education, training, and practice. *AIDS Educ Prev*, 13(6), 561-570.

Chapter Four

Mobilizing the Oral History Archive: HIV/AIDS and the Multimedia Experience in the Classroom and Beyond

Paul Burnett, PhD
Oral History Center, University of California, Berkeley

Abstract

This paper describes the HIV/AIDS oral history archive at the Oral History Center at UC Berkeley and UCSF, the adoption of new archival technology that will form part of the Center's education outreach, and the development of an "Epidemics in History" curriculum for California high schools. Oral histories are excellent primary sources that fulfill the requirements of state standards and guidelines for high school teaching. What follows is an exploration of the nature of oral history, the pedagogical advantages of using oral history in the classroom, the new online audio-video platform being developed at the Oral History Center, the K-16 project to develop guides, curriculum content, sample assignments and project suggestions for Grade 8 and Grade 11, and the ways in which the HIV/AIDS archive can satisfy some the content guidelines for California history-social science standards, and enhance the social-emotional learning and critical thinking skills of high school students.

Storytelling is an ancient form of knowledge transmission, one whose reach has been amplified in recent years by powerful sets of technology platforms that permit the archiving, analysis, recontextualization, and dissemination of first-person historical narratives. At the same time, educational researchers and educators have recognized the potential of storytelling to increase student engagement with history in K-12 schools by integrating first-person narratives into history and social-studies curricula. This paper[1] explores efforts at UC Berkeley and UC San Francisco to bring to students a rich archive on the history of the first encounters with the AIDS epidemic in San Francisco. Following the introduction of the collection of interviews about the early history of the AIDS epidemic in San Francisco, the Oral History Center's plans for reaching students in California high schools will be explored.

In the 1990s, historian Sally Smith Hughes conducted a series of almost three dozen interviews called *The AIDS Epidemic in San Francisco: The Medical Response, 1981-1984,* which are archived at UC Berkeley Oral History Center and the UCSF Library Archives, and hosted online by Calisphere.[2] Hughes wished to focus on medical, scientific and public health improvisations under those early conditions of tremendous uncertainty about the basic nature of the disease, its mechanisms of transmission, and the social, economic, and political context of the infected population. As she interviewed researchers, epidemiologists, and public health officials, however, she recognized there was a significant set of stories in the transformation of nursing care for people living with AIDS and their communities, and raised funds to interview the managers of the AIDS Clinic at San Francisco General Hospital and the founding members of the renowned Ward 5B, which became famous as the so-called San Francisco Model for AIDS care. The final tranche of the interviews was with community physicians with predominantly gay practices who formed a crucial public health early-warning system before the epidemic was fully recognized. All of these interviews are so striking because of the clear understanding that the entire social, political, economic, and cultural landscape needed to be explored in order to render these complex portraits of the epidemic from different perspectives.

This is not to say that the AIDS archives at the Oral History Center or at UCSF are complete. Funding priorities shifted elsewhere, and the tragic story of the epidemic multiplied into a global pandemic. However, these thirty-three interviews are an important beginning. They cover an astonishing range of topics that help us understand more, not only about the early history of the epidemic, but also the history of local, regional, and national politics, including grassroots organizing, civil rights activism, and the public emergence of LGBTQ+ communities; in addition to the history of science, technology, medicine, nursing, and public health. Given these subject areas, this archive has real potential to reach an important audience: students in high school and university. The Oral History Center's embrace of new technology will help us to help students and teachers to meet the requirements of state standards and guidelines for high school teaching. What follows is an exploration of the pedagogical merits of oral history in the classroom, this new online audio-video platform, our outreach generally, our K-16 project to reach out to teachers, and how the HIV/AIDS archive is a great fit for high school and undergraduate teaching.

Oral history, by its nature, can help students to empathize with those who lived at a different time and who had different backgrounds and life experiences from their own. It lends a social-emotional learning component to classes that work with or that conduct their own oral histories. Oral history is an interviewing process that places the person being interviewed—what we refer to as the "narrator"—at center stage. In other types of interviews, with journalists for example, the interview is part of the journalist's larger story. There might be a brief quotation from the interviewee, and the interviewee usually does not have a chance to review what the journalist wrote to verify that the quotation is correct.

The practice of oral history, by contrast, puts the narrator in charge of their part of the project. Interviewer and narrator work together from beginning to end to make sure the recorded story is what the narrator wanted to tell. In other words, the process of working with and doing oral history is itself a process of social-emotional learning, and a model for behavior of young people in a time of relative isolation, misunderstanding, intolerance of difference, and the cultivated mistrust of expertise.

A key question worth exploring with students is about the nature of oral history as evidence. What kind of knowledge is oral history? Does a person's memory of an event have the same truth value as something that was written down at or near the time the event occurred? Is memory reliable? If so, in what sense? Does one person's memories stand up to the official story of how an event unfolded? Is each person's story of equal value? These questions can be discussed with students through examples that are relevant to them. What we at the Oral History Center typically say is that oral history is not about verifying facts. But we would also say that oral history is never *just* a recorded opinion. Oral history is the recording and interpretation of the *facts* of a person's memories, interpreted life experiences, identity, expertise (in whatever form that might take), and way of understanding the world. A memory may ultimately be determined—by researching other historical materials—to be inaccurate, exaggerated, or a complete fabrication. But the fact of the memory is historically significant. Even its difference from other historical evidence can tell you something about what one person, or even groups of people, thought was important enough to remember and recount in a certain way.

The stories we tell each other become an important part of the fabric of our culture, and the variations in stories from person to person reveal the rich texture of human history, and teach us to be humble and careful about how we interpret the past.

On the Oral History Center website, under our "Education" tab, we will host a set of instructions and curricula for teaching epidemics in history, as well as sample assignments and content that will help teachers to tailor their own lesson plans to their specific classes. We have a document about the practice of oral history for high school classes, as well as advice and instructions about how to have students conduct interviews of their own. Although this is, for now, beyond the scope of a discussion of mobilizing the AIDS archive to both preserve and extend our collective memory of epidemics, teaching students how to do oral history can complement their exploration of the archive. Over time, educators may find ways to contribute to the history of HIV/AIDS by having students conduct interviews with survivors of the epidemic. Ultimately, however, the practice of doing and researching oral history share the same basic skill and quality: listening. Students will learn to listen; they will listen to people listening; and they can discuss with their teachers how people listen to one another.

The Oral History Center has also produced content about the history of epidemics for the high school classroom more broadly. Although there are fantastic courses on the history of epidemics, public health, and medicine, they are only taught at a small number of universities. The analytical frameworks of Charles Rosenberg, Steve Epstein, David Barnes, Nancy Tomes, and many other historians helped shape the *First Response* podcast as well as the content for this broader exploration. One goal is to use the history of epidemics to explore larger questions about justice, discrimination, governance, rights, and our shared responsibilities. Even beyond our current context of the COVID-19 pandemic, such questions are evergreen and can support educators' efforts to explore these issues with their students.

Although we have a set of framing documents for teachers, we have also produced instructions to help students navigate our website and work with these oral histories. The Oral History Center currently has over 4,000 long-form oral histories online in transcript form, covering wide swaths of American and world history over the past century. We have digitized audio for many of those interviews going back to the 1950s, and we have video for oral histories recorded after 2004. Under a partnership with the National Parks Service, the OHC completely redesigned its web interface and back end in order to realize new levels of functionality and interactivity. The first phase was to build an advanced, database-driven search engine. We have produced a companion document of how to use the search to find information for most of our collection. The procedure will be a bit different for the AIDS interviews, however, which are hosted on Calisphere.

One solution to this challenge is to roll out a new platform altogether. This second phase in our technological upgrade is an audio-video interface originally developed at the University of Kentucky called the Oral History Metadata Synchronizer. Using "OHMS," students and educators will be able to search the full text and keywords across the entire collection. More importantly, with a YouTube-type video window above the transcript, they will also be able to click over and watch or listen to any point in a stream of an entire interview.

What is remarkable about these technological tools is the degree to which they could facilitate K-12 educators' compliance with standards in reading and science. Under the Common Core State Standards—including most of those that were adopted in place of the Common Core—teachers must "move off the textbook" and engage students with real-world materials, as opposed to literature or poetry, for example. Teachers must not only find this "informational text" on their own, but they also need to be sure that the text and assignment are suitable for a given grade level. To be clear, our oral histories comprise exemplary informational text. They are primary-source documents by witnesses to important historical events and processes; but they are also stories that can engage students directly.

Furthermore, with online oral history recordings–either audio or video– the medium of text as transcripts can be compared with an audio or visual medium, even using the same interview. We will have this capability with our Oral History Metadata Synchronizer, in which the transcripts are synched with the video of the interview. Another criterion for many state educational standards—including the Common Core and its state-adapted variants—is media and digital literacy. Teachers will be able to have students work with different media, and discuss the pros and cons of each. What information is communicated in a video that is difficult or impossible to convey with the printed word? Is working with transcripts easier in some ways than with interview recordings? How can different media be combined to provide compelling secondary narratives? These conceptual questions can be worked through and tested by the students by using the OHMS interface.

The next phase of this work is to develop specific content that will facilitate the use of our collection by educators for Grades 8 and 11, as well as those working in undergraduate history courses. Once we do the groundwork, it is hoped that we can generate the right incentives for a teacher commons that will grow as more teachers use the site, leaving information on their assignments for other teachers to use. We have consulted with the California History-Social Science Project to make sure that the content we develop is relevant to the Grade 11 classroom, which is our pilot class. According to the standards, there are themes that California teachers are supposed to explore in Grade 11: migration, immigration, and globalization; equality and Civil Rights, including the experience of women, African-American, Latin-x, and LGBTQ Americans; community organizations and grassroots reform; technological change; the role of government in society; science in society; political history, and contemporary American society. It should be obvious how the AIDS epidemic archive satisfies most of these guidelines.

For students, we are developing guides and content that will help them learn about historical research practices, how to evaluate different forms of evidence, and how to think critically about the production of their own knowledge across different media: text, photos, audio, and video. So, in this context, how do we help preserve and disseminate memories of the HIV/AIDS epidemic, especially for young people who did not live through this time? What would course content look like, and what do we want them to learn?

One byproduct of our efforts to curate our content for the general public has generated some useful models and content for the classroom. The Oral History Center's efforts to mobilize the AIDS oral history archive — to raise awareness of its existence and to draw in new readers and audiences — began with a new podcast series called *The Berkeley Remix*.[3] Sally Hughes and I both knew that the AIDS archive needed a multi-episode treatment that would reflect at least some of its depth and complexity. We also knew that the podcast could serve both as a teaching tool and as a model for classroom explorations and scaled-down assignments.

For example, the introduction to the first of seven episodes, called "San Francisco," sets up the framework that epidemic disease reveals the fault lines in society, showing differences in access to health care resources, with predictable variations in health outcomes. But a key point of the podcast is that the trajectory of a health crisis is not wholly determined by those fault lines. Epidemics do generate fear and incline people to retreat into familiar patterns of indifference and discrimination; but they also encourage people to rupture those same patterns, and work towards easing the suffering of others and identifying and eliminating its source. The sequence of the episodes walks the listener through the triumphant mood of the gay community in

San Francisco, throwing off the fear and oppression of the dominant culture in the 1970s; the initial fear of both the known and unknown features of the disease; the pre-existing relationships between public health services and the gay community's own mobilization around infectious diseases; the challenge to the fragile trust developed between the state and this community; the struggle for resources to research and fight the disease in a context of indifference to a marginalized community; and the provisional triumph of a new, more humane way of caring for and treating patients in hospitals and clinics. That list by itself may not be very compelling. But this two-and-a-half hours' worth of podcasts help to frame a large archive that might otherwise be daunting to anyone but a specialist researcher. Like many multimedia presentations, however, there is also a strong affective component. This is difficult, emotional material, and the audio of the interviews gives audiences a more direct window on the worlds of those who survived the epidemic, as well as those who didn't.

When we put this podcast together with our new OHMS system and sample curriculum content, students and educators will soon be able to work with the entire digitized audio from this archive. In addition, during the spring semester, we worked with four undergraduate students at UC Berkeley to develop a set of model assignments using different media that would be scaled to a grade-eleven assignment: a twitter thread, a student forum, an infographic, and a traditional essay. They also wrote accompanying process documents detailing how they found information through the advanced search. We soon hope to add more multimedia examples of what students can do once the AIDS interviews are completely prepared for the OHMS platform. We also developed content, lesson plans, and resources for four additional projects that extend the themes of the *First Response* podcast. With this modeled content, user guides, and grade-level-specific assignments, we want students to think critically about the following:

- How are values and cultural biases built into the structure of institutions, either actively or passively?
- How do excluded and heretofore invisible communities empower themselves and gain access to resources?
- To what extent are science, technology, medicine, and disease social phenomena that are subject to other social, political, and economic forces?
- What values drive people to reach across boundaries of difference to improve the lives of both specific groups and the general public?

In other words, the AIDS archive is not dry, historical source material; it is a vehicle for exploring philosophical, epistemological, and political issues about how we understand and present the past to others.

We want students to reflect of the nature of archives themselves in doing this work. Historians and philosophers have long pointed out that the first step in history-making is what gets included in the archive in the first place. For example, as Sally pointed out, the AIDS oral history project focused on the early years of the epidemic: research and treatment for a gay, but largely white, male population. Historian Eleanor Naiman, who has been working with us at the Center, is making use of both the archive at UCSF and her own oral history interviews to uncover a different facet of the epidemic. She is analyzing the experiences of HIV-positive women activists in San Francisco in a time-frame after our oral history archive: from the late 1980s until the mid-1990s. By adding such material to our archives, we can broaden our questions, not only about who was affected by the disease, but also about how disease is framed by choices we make as recorders of history. Not only is disease political, but so is the archive itself. That is something we want young people to absorb as they question the narratives that have been handed to them, and as they begin to think about defining their own voices by listening to those of others.

Finally, as students move beyond both the textbook and the standard historical essay in their assignments, we want them to pay careful attention to the differences among kinds of historical evidence and media, and to reflect on the power of each medium to help readers and audiences make meaning from history. Ultimately, this means that we also need to help both educators and students with making their own versions of this history. This is what our new curriculum content will facilitate, including sample syllabi for undergraduate courses, sequenced assignments for Grades 8 and 11 that teach students how to use this archive, how to access other archival resources, especially UCSF's digital collections, and eventually how to create multimedia content. For example, students could make a multimedia blog, or even a "live," scaled-down version of a podcast using the OHMS interface. For teachers, we plan to marshal secondary resources to help them with background on the history of the epidemic.

Our answer to the question of sustaining the memory of those who encountered and fought the epidemic is to draw on the powerful, emotional aspects of this multimedia archive, to identify the needs of prospective audiences, especially students and educators in our school, and to help them learn, and feel, something about this important part of modern US history. Watch the Oral History Center main page for the "Epidemics in History" coming in August, 2020.[4]

Endnotes

1. A version of this paper was delivered at the "Memory Lives On" Symposium, held at UCSF on Oct. 5 2019, by Roger Eardley-Pryor, Sally Smith Hughes, and Eleanor Naiman.
2. The interviews are hosted online on Calisphere, but are accessible through the Oral History Center project page - https://www.lib.berkeley.edu/libraries/bancroft-library/oral-history-center/projects/aids and search page: https://www.lib.berkeley.edu/libraries/bancroft-library/oral-history-center/advanced-search-form, as well as through the UCSF Library page: https://www.library.ucsf.edu/archives/aids/oral-history-project/. Retrieved June 17, 2020.
3. Paul Burnett, "First Response: AIDS and Community in San Francisco," *The Berkeley Remix*. Podcast. Season 3. December, 2018. ucblib.link/BRS3. Retrieved June 16, 2020.
4. To check in on progress on this work, click on the "Education" tab of the Oral History Center website: https://www.lib.berkeley.edu/libraries/bancroft-library/oral-history-center

References

Burnett, Paul. (2018). "First Response: AIDS and Community in San Francisco," *The Berkeley Remix*. Podcast. Season 3. ucblib.link/BRS3. Retrieved June 16, 2020.

Epstein, Steven. (1998). *Impure Science: AIDS, Activism, and the Politics of Knowledge*. Berkeley: University of California Press.

Rosenberg, Charles. (1962). *The Cholera Years: The United States in 1832, 1849, and 1866*. Chicago: University of Chicago Press.

___. (1992). *Explaining Epidemics and other Studies in the History of Medicine*. New York: Cambridge University Press.

Tomes, Nancy. (1991). "Oral History in the History of Medicine." *Journal of American History*. 78 (No.2), 607-17.

___. (2000). "The Making of a Germ Panic, Then and Now." *American Journal of Public Health*. 90 (No.2), 191-98.

Chapter Five

Obituary Parlor Games: Collecting and Analyzing Obituaries as Sources for Understanding the AIDS Epidemic

Elizabeth Alice Clement, PhD
Department of History, University of Utah

This essay is a meditation on the value of obituaries as a source for understanding the AIDS epidemic in the United States. I begin with the ethical issues of archiving AIDS obituaries and the importance of knowing their form and provenance when using them. I then address the patterns I have found when running statistical analyses of AIDS obituaries from Utah. These analyses tell us a great deal about the choices people made about disclosing an AIDS diagnosis and thus how visible the epidemic was to the general newspaper-reading population in a conservative place like Utah. They also reveal shifts in the understanding of the place of queer people in the American family in the 1980s and 1990s that are not visible through any other sources. I conclude with a discussion of what I know about how and why gay people in Utah read and collected obituaries. I demonstrate that doing so came to constitute its own death ritual for a community reeling from catastrophic loss. As such, this paper traces the way one kind of death ritual, the obituary, catalyzed other death rituals, facilitating people's ability to process and cope with grief.[1]

I must begin with a caveat. My data and conclusions come from the epidemic in Utah, a majority white, politically conservative state in the Rocky Mountains dominated by the Mormon church. While Utah had non-gay sources of transmission, the epidemic here overwhelmingly struck white men who had sex with men, a majority of whom identified as gay.[2] Because the non-white population of Utah was so small in the 1980s and 1990s and because our patterns of drug-use were different, Utah did not experience the epidemic among African American and Latinx folks that occurred in the

Northeast and coastal West and that is now ravaging the American South. That said, like many other places, African Americans and Latinx folks were and are overrepresented relative to their percentage in the population. This does not make our collection of obituaries unimportant, but it does limit the scope of what my analysis can say about the HIV epidemic as it occurred in other, more diverse places.

While I argue that collecting and analyzing obituaries should be a priority for all AIDS related archives, doing so raises ethical concerns that must be thoughtfully addressed. The majority of AIDS obituaries in Utah, and in my estimation nationwide, do not mention AIDS at all. Which is to say, families and individuals consistently chose NOT to be open about what many at the time saw as a shameful identity (gayness) and a shameful death (from AIDS). If the archive in question is an AIDS archive, simply placing obituaries in it clearly identifies them as AIDS dead. This is problematic for two reasons. First, it reveals medical information. However, obituaries are published and thus do not fall under HIPAA (the Health Insurance Portability and Accountability Act of 1996.)[3] As a result, obituaries do not pose legal issues for archives. But if we agree that the spirit animating HIPAA is that all people have the right to medical privacy, then we should live by HIPAA guidelines even if we work in an archive and not a hospital. Second, outing people with AIDS violates long-standing gay community ethical norms. The American gay community has long believed that same-sex attracted people have the right to choose whether to disclose their sexuality to a hostile world. Although not everyone who died of AIDS identified as gay, the issues of AIDS stigma remain the same regardless of the route of transmission. Gay community norms should be honored by archives and researchers when considering the privacy of the AIDS dead.

However, most archives already employ restrictions to control sensitive materials. In the 1990s, I applied for and received permission to use prison records held by the New York State Archives. The records I used contained intimate details about people who might have been alive. As a condition of having access to these files I agreed to use ethnically-appropriate pseudonyms and mask any identifying biographical information. I see no reason why archives should not employ similar restrictions for obituaries in AIDS collections. Further, when I used similar files at the New York Public Library, the restrictions on the Women's Prison Association (WPA) papers required that I apply to the organization directly. This added level of bureaucracy gave the WPA the ability to assess my goals as a researcher. As part of the creation of the University of Utah's "Ries/Snyder HIV Archive," we are currently developing similar protocols. The Utah AIDS Foundation (UAF) has asked to have final say over whether researchers may use the restricted portions of their papers. Obviously, such restrictions must detail what to do in case the organization generating the files ceases operation. Sadly, in the case of AIDS related work, this seems unlikely until such time as the United States provides universal healthcare to its population and ends the epidemic. Collecting AIDS obituaries presents ethical concerns for archives, but these are not insurmountable. Thoughtful discussions with donating agencies and carefully written restrictions can easily resolve these concerns.

When it comes to using obituaries as historical sources, researchers must understand how they are produced, where they were published and who wrote them. In the nineteenth-century newspapers only published obituaries of public figures. But in twentieth century, like a lot of things, obituaries in America democratized.[4] By the time the AIDS crisis broke, obituaries functioned more to let the community know that someone had died than to memorialize someone of public prominence. In Utah, and around the country, funeral homes provided templates from which mourners could craft obituaries. Although not everyone used these templates, they did shape the information families gave as well as the general order in which it appeared. This is why so many obituaries seem so similar. Except for people like Les Stewart, who wrote, "my picture on this page means that I have finally died," it is impossible to know who wrote any given obituary.[5] However, my oral history data indicates that natal kin, and not gay kin or the dead themselves, wrote the majority of Utah's AIDS obituaries.[6]

Most obituaries offer the same basic biographical data, what scholar Janice Hume refers to as "four framing categories": "name and occupation of the deceased, cause of death, personal attributes of the deceased, and funeral arrangements."[7] The vast majority of Utah obituaries also refer to the dates and places of birth and death. Obituaries often solicit donations, either to a fund related to the cause of death: "in lieu of flowers make donations to American Cancer Society," or a cause or organization important to the deceased: "in lieu of flowers make donations to the Pioneer Theater Company." Finally, most obituaries have a "kinship" sentence, also known as the "survived by" sentence. The kinship sentence ostensibly informs the reader which family members who survive the dead. They identify for the public who is bereaved by this death, and thus who is deserving of community support in their grief.[8]

It is also important to know which newspapers published the obituaries. The way people clip obituaries can make this identification difficult. I have been able to address this problem because I know who collected the obituaries

I use, and so could ask. With AIDS obituaries the issue of mainstream papers versus gay papers really matters. Gay papers would be much more likely to be open about issues like death from AIDS and gayness itself than mainstream papers, even those published in the same geographical area. Obituaries published in mainstream papers are also more likely to be written by natal kin, while lovers and gay kin author more, if not all, of those published in gay papers. Horacio Roque Ramirez analyzed the Latinx obituaries published in San Francisco's gay paper, the *Bay Area Reporter* (*BAR*), for what they can tell us about the lives of gay Latinx men and their experiences in the epidemic.[9] As we will see, Ramirez found rates of references to AIDS as a cause of death significantly higher than those from Utah, but it is impossible to know whether that is because he analyzed a gay paper or because San Francisco is a much more liberal place than Utah. In all likelihood, it is a combination of both.

Although Utah generally follows practices common in the rest of the United States, as in all local histories, there are some interesting variations. Utah may actually produce more obituaries per person than other places because of the dominance of The Church of Jesus Christ of Latter-day Saints (Mormon Church). *The General Handbook of Instruction*, a guide used by the lay bishops who run day to day operations in local wards, provides extensive instructions as to how bishops should help families with death rituals. These include the directive that bishops to "see that the newspapers are properly notified, ensuring that a complete and accurate obituary is filed."[10] The religious importance of genealogy to Mormons undoubtedly drives these instructions. The two largest papers in Utah, the *Salt Lake Tribune* and the *Deseret News* shared obituaries, which meant that a death notice placed in one paper would be printed in the other.[11] Knowing that makes it easier for me to estimate the reach of the obituaries I have, because I can reasonably assume that most people in the state who read obituaries would have had access to the same information, regardless of which paper they read.

Around the country in the 1980s and 1990s obituaries in mainstream papers consistently failed to mention the cause of death as AIDS, much less acknowledge the homosexuality of gay people with AIDS who had died. In part this may have stemmed from historical conventions in the genre that allow for discretion around shameful issues like extramarital affairs, criminal behavior or, in the past, divorce.[12] Obituaries have always balanced uneasily between the desire to valorize the dead and the impulse to be true to them. However, AIDS hit at precisely the moment when the "shame" of homosexuality had become a subject of intense debate. Post-Stonewall, gay people argued that there was nothing shameful about homosexuality and that it should not be hidden. Some straight people agreed, others fiercely disagreed, while still others probably ignored these discussions altogether. But it is clear that not mentioning AIDS or homosexuality in obituaries, especially given the importance of "coming out" to the gay community in the 1980s and 1990s, cannot be seen as quite the same as refusing to discuss divorce or an extramarital affair. Gay liberation mobilized coming out as a political strategy, which made AIDS obituaries political texts.

Literary critic Dagmawi Woubshet provides a fascinating example of choices newspapers made around whether to reveal AIDS and homosexuality in obituaries. He compares two 1983 obituaries for musician Paul Jacobs, one from the *New York Times* and the other from the gay-run *New York Native*. Touting his accomplishments as a composer, the *New York Times* did not mention his lover of twenty-two years nor his cause of death as AIDS. The *New York Native* obituary not only noted these facts but chastised the *Times*, caustically remarking, "although the *New York Times* obituary made no mention of his sexual orientation and attributed his death to 'a long illness,' Mr. Jacobs was an openly gay man who wanted the nature of his illness to be a matter of public record."[13] Obituaries from the most liberal cities routinely re-closeted men who had been out for years and who had wanted their deaths from AIDS to be marked to make the epidemic more visible. Not listing AIDS as the cause of death masked the severity of the epidemic, making it harder mobilize political pressure on the government to dedicate resources to end it.

As Woubshet demonstrates, the founding of ACT UP in New York City in 1987 accelerated the political deployment of death rituals, including obituaries. ACT UP's famous "silence equals death" slogan—rendered on posters, stickers, and tee-shirts—encouraged people to be out about their HIV status, and if they were gay, their homosexuality. Responding to this call, many of the dying began to insist that their obituaries acknowledge AIDS as the cause of death. ACT UP's 1991 "Clip and Mail AIDS Obits" campaign asked people "around the country" to send obituaries of the AIDS dead to President Bush and First Lady Barbara Bush to pressure them to increase their advocacy for AIDS related causes.[14] Highlighting the commonness of hiding the AIDS dead in death notices, ACT UP recommended that if the obituary did not mention AIDS that protestors should annotate it.[15] Although ACT UP chapters and actions tended to be concentrated in big liberal cities like New York and San Francisco, anyone could participate in the "Clip and Mail" campaign. While Salt Lake City had an AIDS ward and an AIDS Service Organization (UAF), it did not have an ACT UP chapter. But people involved in AIDS here followed ACT UP's actions carefully, even as they also felt that its confrontational style would be counterproductive in such a conservative place.[16] My oral histories indicate that people with AIDS in Utah discussed the politics of mentioning AIDS in their death notices. Obituaries that referenced AIDS began appearing in Salt Lake's newspapers by the late 1980s. This would have been before the "Clip and Mail" campaign, but after ACT UP introduced "silence equals death" as a slogan. As conservative and religious as Utah was, gay people here participated in national conversations about the political nature of the AIDS epidemic and the importance of visibility to both gay civil rights and AIDS.

I have two datasets of AIDS obituaries for Utah. Their provenance, who gathered them and what that person's position relative to the epidemic was, is crucial for understanding what they can tell us. The first set come from Maggie Snyder's scrapbooks. Snyder worked first as a nurse on the state's only AIDS ward and then as the physician's assistant to Doctor Ries, the only doctor in the state treating people with AIDS for the first decade of the epidemic. Snyder collected 285 obituaries between 1991 and 2009. Because Ries and Snyder cared for upwards of 90% of Utah's AIDS caseload between 1987 and 2009, Snyder's obituaries provide an invaluable resource for tracking how open people were about AIDS and thus, how visible AIDS actually was to the people of Utah. The Snyder collection is probably unique. Health care providers in, say, San Francisco, undoubtedly clipped obituaries. But they would not have been the only medical professionals treating people with AIDS in the city, much less in the state of California. The epidemic in places like San Francisco and New York grew too big too quickly for anyone to be able to create the kind of birds-eye view of AIDS in Utah that Snyder produced.

Ben Williams collected the second set of 238 obituaries from 1989 to 1999.[17] An out gay man, Williams has functioned as an informal historian of Salt Lake's gay community for the last forty years. Williams knew–or knew of– many of the gay men who died in the epidemic. Unlike Snyder, his information would have been concentrated in Salt Lake. He would have known little about the epidemic in smaller cities like Logan or Ogden, or in rural areas. He also would have been less aware of people with AIDS who did not identify as gay. In Utah that was hemophiliacs, closeted same-sex attracted men and injection drug users. Those obituaries, Williams would have missed. The kind of collecting Williams did was very common. Around the country people close to the epidemic clipped and saved obituaries of lovers, friends, co-workers and at times, acquaintances. Both Snyder and Williams mostly relied on the *Salt Lake Tribune* for their obituaries, though there are a smattering from Salt

Lake's gay paper, the *Pillar*.[18]

Like obituaries in mainstream papers nationwide, the majority of obituaries of Utah's AIDS dead did not mention AIDS. In the Snyder dataset, only 24.2% of the obituaries list the cause of death as AIDS, for the Williams that number is 39.5%. If you combine the number of people who gave AIDS as a cause of death with the people who asked for donations to an AIDS Service Organization (ASO), those numbers rise to 31.6% and 48.3% respectively. Because people often ask for donations related to the disease that caused their death and because AIDS was so stigmatized, it seems reasonable to assume that the families who wrote these obituaries deliberately risked the stigma of AIDS in order to encourage donations to ASOs. People with AIDS in Utah knew that neither the federal government or their own state government was providing resources to fund research, prevention, or care. In a time of profound underfunding of all AIDS related services, the authors of these obituaries sacrificed family privacy and reputation to support organizations they knew provided crucial services. But even when I include donations, the number of people mentioning AIDS does not reach 50%, indicating the strength of that stigma and its attendant shame. This is particularly ironic given the directive in the *General Handbook of Instruction* that bishops help families file "complete and accurate obituary."[19] LDS families published obituaries for their AIDS dead, but clearly bishops failed to make them either "complete" or "accurate."

The different levels of knowledge Snyder and Williams had about the epidemic explain the gap in their numbers. Snyder knew everyone being treated for AIDS, and as a result, her obituaries captured more of both the non-gay AIDS related deaths and those of closeted men. Williams' dataset, on the other hand, oversampled for out gay men like himself. When thinking about this in terms of the visibility of AIDS, the Snyder numbers tell us that people reading the obituaries in *Salt Lake Tribune* could only see about one third of the epidemic in the state. This mattered because hiding AIDS made the epidemic seem smaller and the losses less devastating. The men in Williams' dataset were much more likely to identify as gay and as a result to interpret the failure of the government to respond to AIDS as a political issue. As ACT UP's actions made national news, many of these men would have considered death rituals an appropriate place to make a political statement about AIDS. For example, Bryant Park died in 1994 at the age of 36. His obituary stated, "Bryant's wish is that people will become aware and learn about HIV and AIDS because too many people are dying from this disease" and asked that donations be made to the Utah AIDS Foundation "to help support those with AIDS."[20] Others used obituaries to reject the shame attached to AIDS and homosexuality. As Robert Dean Johnson's 1994 obituary stated, "Robert was a proud gay man, he loved life and was loved by many. He will be greatly missed." Robert was 34 when he died.[21] These death notices make it clear that some people with AIDS in Utah shared ACT UP's sense that obituaries could and should be political. But AIDS as a cause of death still appeared less than 40% of the time. Since there are no statistical comparisons available for larger more liberal cities, it is hard to know whether Utah's numbers are similar, or if they are low because Utah is such a conservative place.

In contrast to the Utah numbers of 31.6% and 48.3%, Horacio Roque Ramirez's analysis of Latinx obituaries in San Francisco's gay paper found "more than two-thirds...made direct reference to AIDS-related complications."[22] He notes that the high percentage of obituaries mentioning AIDS reflects the fact that "the *BAR* early on emerged as the city's 'informal' public record of how the disease was progressing in the gay community."[23] This might distinguish the *BAR* even from gay papers in other cities, which may not have seen mentioning AIDS in their obituaries as critical to their mission. Only an 18% difference separates the AIDS obituaries in the *BAR* and those from the Utah papers Ben Williams read. Given the conservative and deeply religious culture in Utah, I found this surprising. It indicates out-gay people in conservative places followed and participated in national gay conversations about AIDS. It also shows that many more of them than we might expect agreed that making AIDS more visible, even in such a hostile place, was crucial to the fight against the disease. Future scholars should explore whether these differences derive from in the fact that the *BAR* is a gay paper, or whether the *San Francisco Chronicle* had significantly higher references to AIDS as well, which would reflect regional and political differences.

Beyond the visibility of AIDS, the Utah obituaries also indicate the degree to which families had begun to acknowledge (and thus, for the audience reading, to see) gay people in their families and communities. Using the "kinship sentence" has allowed me to track the numbers of families that acknowledged lovers as kin. This in turn makes it possible to see the progress we, as queer people made in making homosexuality visible within the heart of the American family during the 1980s and 1990s. For context, Gallup conducted a poll in 1983 that found that only 24% of Americans said they had a gay "friend or acquaintance."[24] Given how hard gay activists pushed "coming out" as a strategy of political empowerment in the wake of the 1969 Stonewall uprising, that is a shockingly low number. The phrasing is also interesting. The survey did not even ask if respondents had family who were gay. Nor can we know, if it had asked about family, whether that number would go up or down. Americans assume that we know our family better than we know friends, but in the case of homosexuality, historically that has tended not to be true. Gay people, especially in the 1970s and 1980s would come out to friends first, usually other gay people, and then to peer-aged kin like siblings. As a result, older Americans in the 1980s would be less likely to know that they had gay kin, while younger Americans might be more likely. Region, religion and political affiliation would also matter. People born and raised in liberal places and faith traditions would be more likely to know they had gay kin than those raised in places like Utah. But 24% works as a good baseline for Americans' awareness of homosexuality. AIDS obituaries provide a fascinating window into the degree to which that knowledge and public recognition of it shifted because of AIDS.

In the Snyder dataset, 22.8% of obituaries mentioned someone in the kinship sentence who can be interpreted as a long-term lover. Not surprisingly, in the Williams data the percentage of lovers mentioned was higher, 35.3%. However, I argue that even Snyder's 22.8% number is remarkably high. As both the obituaries and my oral histories attest, many people's lovers had already passed away from AIDS. Other people were simply un-partnered when they died. Given that, the Snyder number of 22.8% almost matches Gallup's 24%. The higher Williams number, again, reflects his oversampling for out gay men who were more likely to insist that their lovers be included. These men's families, who were still more likely to write the obituary than gay kin, may also have become accustomed to seeing the lovers as part of the family. As I have argued elsewhere, joint caregiving for people with AIDS brought families of origin and out gay people into intimate contact with each other, often in gay controlled spaces like a couple's home, which accelerated straight acknowledgement of gay people as family.[25]

Unlike the issue of people willing to print the cause of death as AIDS, we have no comparative data to help contextualize the mention of lovers in the kinship sentence. Ramirez did not provide percentages for lovers listed in the *BAR* obituaries, though he did note that when authors mentioned them, they "marked same-sex (gay) relationships." Even if he had, though, as a gay paper, *BAR* would have received far more obituaries that acknowledged gay kin than Utah's mainstream papers. We also lack historical comparisons. Given the level of closeting before AIDS, it seems unlikely that families in the 1960s or 1970s would have included information about a lover. Some families would not have known the lover, others may have accepted the fiction that the lover was a "roommate." And, of course, in the 1960s and 1970s, there would have been far fewer gay deaths and less political pressure from gay people themselves to mark homosexuality in an obituary. The data from Utah demonstrates the movement of gay people into the kinship sentence and thus the acknowledgement on the part of the straight kin who wrote these obituaries, that gay people were kin.

In both datasets families used similar terms to describe lovers and did so in about the same proportion. In the Snyder obituaries, for example, the most common phrases used to describe lovers were "long-time companion" at 38.5%, "special" or "dear" friend at 29.2%, partner at 24.6% and lover at 7.7%. In the Williams dataset, "friend" modified in various ways proved the most popular at 39.8%, followed by companion at 34.9%, partner at 9.6% and lover at 1.2%. The Williams data also had the unambiguous term "mate," usually modified with "life" or "soul" in 7.2% of mentions, a term absent from the Snyder dataset. The most significant difference lay in the tiny proportion (7.2%) of obituaries in the Williams data set that referred to "husband" or "spouse," also completely missing from the Sndyer.

The language used to describe gay partners reflects the contested nature of gay membership in straight families. First, the absence of "husband" or "spouse" in the Snyder, and its tiny percentage in the Williams, indicates just how far we were from gay marriage even as late as the 1990s. Gay marriage burst into the American popular consciousness when Hawaii's Supreme Court ruled in 1993 in *Baehr v. Lewin* that denial of marriage "constituted discrimination based on sex."[26] This galvanized a conservative backlash intended to preempt any action by courts or liberal states to give gay people access to marriage. That only 7.2 % of obituaries in the openly-gay dominated Williams data indicates that even gay people had trouble imagining gay marriage. It also shows how many families could not make the mental leap to acknowledge that gay lovers might be similar—either emotionally or in terms of caregiving labor—to spouses. But the small number of references to 'husband" can be balanced by how easy to read euphemisms like "long-time companion," "partner" and "mate" turned up even in the Snyder dataset. "Friend" is ambiguous; many of us do have close "friends" who are not lovers. But the word "friend" usually came with other clarifying language like "special" or combined with other marking words as in "best friend and companion" that made the meaning clear.[27] These euphemisms feel so formulaic that they out people, even when families obviously wanted the language to be discrete. And of course, as the legal next of kin, families could ignore lovers. This makes including a romantic partner a deliberate choice to acknowledge a gay relationship remarkable, even as it remained cloaked in the language of the closet. Finally, the scarcity of the term "lover" reflects the ways that families, and sometimes gay people themselves, de-sexualized homosexuality in public documents, even as they acknowledged it. Lover just comes too close to sex to make it comfortable in an obituary.

The issue of the location of lovers in the kinship sentence also provides crucial information about the place gay people held in the American family. Here, knowing something about obituaries as a literary form is helpful. Traditionally, if someone marries, their spouse is listed first in the kinship sentence, followed by children and then parents and siblings. If they have not married, the kinship sentence begins with parents, and then follows a similar hierarchy of siblings, cousins and other natal kin.[28] Thus, the place where families mention lovers can function as a measure of their understanding of the level of relatedness. By mentioning a same-sex lover at all, the obituary writer signals that this family had a gay person in it—in the form of the deceased himself. At the same time, referencing a lover validates and makes visible the families that gay people formed. Stanley Dee Nelson's 1994 obituary (he died at 31) began the kinship sentence with "his companion, Michael Cutler," followed by his mother. David Decker Freezy Frost drafted his own 1992 obituary when he died at 34. He placed his current lover in the spouse position, followed by his parents. "I lived a full and wonderful life with my life mate, Michael Ray Bohney," he wrote, "and was preceded in death by Roger [past lover] in 1989."[30] Placing a lover first in the kinship sentence would be a radical move in the 1990s because it gestured towards marriage. It literally placed the lover in the position of spouse, even if the couple could not marry. This, I argue, marks a profound shift in American understandings of family, even in the absence the mechanisms to create family under the law. Placing the lover last relegates them to the position of ancillary kin like cousins, but even that marks a movement towards publicly acknowledging gay people as kin.

On the question of what my data says about where lovers get placed in the kinship sentence, the evidence is interestingly mixed. In both datasets, an almost equal number of obituaries place the lover in the beginning, middle, or end of the kinship sentence. In the Snyder dataset 33.9% of lovers ended up in the "spouse" position. This is close to 32.1% in the Williams. Similarly, 30.8% of the Snyder obituaries placed the lovers at the end, which relegates lovers to the position of more distant kin. For the Williams obituaries the number was 28.6%. Families placed 34.5% of lovers in the middle in the Snyder and 39.3% in the Williams. These mixed results indicate that while these obituary writers did see lovers as some kind of kin, families in Utah did not agree on what degree of kinship gay lovers represented. Further, the similarities of those numbers indicate that being out about homosexuality (as more men in the Williams would have been), did not make a difference in where families positioned them. While a third of families clearly positioned them as spouses, the majority mixed them in with kin of varying degrees of relatedness. Overall, these obituaries indicate that, even in conservative and deeply religious Utah, AIDS began to shift understandings of gay people's relationship to family. Rather than seen as a danger to the American family, as they had been since the sex-crime panics of the 1950s, Utah's AIDS obituaries reflect gay people moving into families, though in uneven and inconsistent ways.[31]

Two obituaries pushed the politics of the kinship sentence even further. Steven Scott Markland died at age 34 in 1994. Although it is not clear who wrote his obituary, the kinship sentence began with his parents but concluded with the loss of "many, many friends to AIDS."[32] By positioning them in the kinship sentence, Markland's "many, many friends" became, by the conventions of obituaries, kin. Les Stewart wrote his own 1996 obituary when he died at age 51. In a standard variation on the kinship sentence, he discussed the kin who died before him: "I am preceded in death by my grandparents, a nephew, Cameron Meyers and 170,000 people in this nation who have died of AIDS, many of them brave and resilient souls, who have fought against impossible medical and numbing social odds." He continued, "In a strange way, I am proud to be numbered among such incredible people."[33] Placing "170,000" AIDS dead in the kinship sentence extended gay understandings of "chosen family" to cover not just other queer people, but the entirety of the AIDS dead. Obituaries, then, could be a place to radically expand the membership in the American family away from biological or legal ties and towards other affinities—affinities of queerness, oppression and disease.

Like many around the nation, gay people close to the epidemic in Utah read the obituaries carefully and played what novelist Armistead Maupin referred to as "obituary parlor games." In *Sure of You*, the sixth of Maupin's best-selling *Tales of the City* series, the main character Michael Toliver's lover has a tantrum about the ways prominent gay men in San Francisco hid their AIDS diagnoses. In the scene, an obituary attributing death to "liver cancer" touched off Thack's wrath. "For the past few years Thack had made a parlor game out of spotting the secret AIDS deaths in the obituary columns," Maupin wrote, "Given the age of the deceased, the absence of a spouse, and certain telltale occupational data, he would draw his own conclusions and fly into a towering rage." "'Notice how they called him flamboyant? How's that for a code word?'" Thack seethed, "How dare he act ashamed? Who does he think he's fooling anyway?" When Michael tried to soothe Thack and maintain respect for the dead, Thack expressed the politics beneath his anger. "This is why people don't give a shit about AIDS!" he shouted, "Because cowardly pricks like this make it seem like it's not really happening!"[34]

In Utah, my narrators used the same criteria as Thack to look for the hidden AIDS obituaries. As Rick Pace described, "when you see a twenty-year old passing away and not married, it was pretty obvious."[35] Like Thack, references to "cancer," tipped people off, as did phrases like "died of a lingering illness."[36] Or, as Patty Reagan noted, "you saw a single man, twenty-two years old, who died of pneumonia. We all knew."[37] However, Pace said biggest clue when playing obituary parlor games in Utah turned out to be local. Families thanked Dr. Ries, Maggie Snyder and the nuns of the Holy Cross for their tireless care. "Every morning I would get up and read the… obituary page" Pace recalled, "they'd always thank Dr. Ries… it was always there."[38] By 1994 the *Salt Lake Tribune* actually ran an article on AIDS titled "Thank You Dr. Kristen Ries and Maggie." The first line of the story read "'The family wishes to thank Dr. Kristen Ries and Maggie' is a familiar line to Utahns who read obituaries. The thanks come from those who have lost a son, a brother, a friend to AIDS."[39] Thanking Ries acknowledged her hard work and compassion. But it also served as a barely coded reference for any person following the epidemic closely. Everybody in the gay community knew Ries was the only doctor who treated people with AIDS in the state. In a poignant variation on "for a good time call," Ries' name was scrawled on the bathroom walls of Salt Lake's gay disco, the Sun Tavern.[40] But straight people, most of whom were not tracking the epidemic carefully, would have missed the reference. That made thanking Ries safe for families, even as they also hid precisely what it was that Ries had helped them with.

However, the Snyder and Williams datasets complicate Pace's memory in ways that reveal both the value of obituaries as a source and the way that triangulating data, that is, combining data from different sources, produces more accurate analysis and information. While some obituaries that did not list AIDS as the cause of death thanked Ries and Snyder, it was far more common for people who were open about dying from AIDS to do so. Of the obituaries that mention Dr. Ries, 42.9% in the Snyder and 25.6% in the Williams hid their AIDS diagnosis. Using Pace's local clue, somewhere between a quarter (Williams' 25.6%) and half (Snyder's 42.9%) of the epidemic became visible for those who knew to look for Ries' name. Rick Pace was right when he said that thanking Ries revealed more of the epidemic than the other clues used in obituary parlor games. But he was wrong when he asserted that "it was always there." Dr. Ries received far more public gratitude from people who had already made the political commitment to openly discuss AIDS in an obituary.

Comparing my oral histories to Maupin's description reveals important differences that might reflect Maupin's imagination, but might represent regional variations in the ways gay people experienced and interpreted obituaries. Published in 1989, almost a decade into the crisis, Maupin's *Sure of You* assumes that closeted gay men chose not to list AIDS because they were ashamed of their homosexuality and wanted to protect their posthumous reputations. While that undoubtedly happened in Utah, my narrators had a very different interpretation. My oral histories indicate that most gay people in Utah assumed that families, and not gay people, wrote obituaries. As Maggie Snyder said, "you have to remember, it's not the person that writes the obituary, it's the family."[41] Ben Williams agreed adding that natal kin "didn't want that disgrace associated with their families."[42] In Utah, and perhaps in other conservative places, gay people who played obituary parlor games did not interpret these obituaries as internalized homophobia. Living and writing in the much more gay friendly context of San Francisco, Maupin may have had more experience with men who could direct their own death rituals. After all, most gay people in San Francisco moved there and thus did not live near natal kin. Staying in San Francisco for care rather than going home to die would have shaped their ability to control what happened after their death. It also may have strengthened partner and friends' ability to run rituals according to the wishes of the dead. Undoubtedly some natal kin still swooped in from afar to big cities to collect inheritance and dispose of bodies. In fact, we know from memoirs like Amy Hoffman's *Hospital Time*, that this happened all the time.[43] But overall, the position of gay kin in liberal San Francisco would have been stronger and easier to enforce both culturally, and by the early 1990s, in the courts.

The emotional response of my narrators also differed significantly from Maupin's account. I only have one example of a narrator who, like the fictional Thack, went into "a towering rage." David Andreason is still angry. As he fumed in his interview, "these gay people who struggled with AIDS and died, without the support of their families, having the added insult in their obituary of having their entire life erased. You can't even list what they died of." "That's just been a very big part of our history," he continued, "being at the mercy of the straight community, and always [needing to] make it so they're comfortable."[44] Here Andreason linked AIDS to a subtle yet totalizing form of homophobia that required gayness be invisible in public. Angry about the fact that even as they suffered and died, gay people's lives would be "erased" not for a noble cause, but just to make heterosexuals "comfortable" transformed his grief into rage. As Deborah Gould argues in *Moving Politics*, her pioneering work on ACT UP, anger and rage became the animating feature of ACT UP and the more confrontational gay politics of the late 1980s and early 1990s.[45] Andreason, even as he eschewed ACT UP's politics, and he explicitly did, clearly shared its rage.

But, for most people, "obituary parlor games" evoked the much more straight-forward reaction of grief and loss. "Every day I'd pick up the newspaper and go to the obituary column and there'd be two or three," bartender Nikki Boyer said, "Every day. Every day it was. I have no men friends my age. They're all gone. That whole generation died off."[46] Her repetition of "day" emphasizes the mundane experience of AIDS deaths at the height of the epidemic. Her personal losses "I have no men friends my age" became a nationwide experience as a "whole generation died off." The combination of daily and unimaginable marked gay grief in the era of AIDS. It was ordinary and daily, but also almost unimaginably catastrophic. Of course grief and anger are not mutually exclusive. Although he spoke in the context of ACT UP, and not obituaries, Joe Munsey discussed both grief and rage in the same breath when he remembered his time with ACT UP New York in the late 1980s. As Munsey explained, he joined ACT UP "because I was angry and what kept me going through the day was anger… it helped me get to a place where I could come back with anger instead of shame." "But the grief was also there," he continued, "it was like I was blaming society for killing my husband, for killing my best friend, [because] we were just watching people drop like flies all around us."[47] Munsey's anger protected him from shame, but the grief remained constant.

Most people played obituary parlor games at home, but those working in AIDS also used the information to keep track of their patients. As Maggie Snyder noted "in those days we watched the obituaries all the time."[48] The Utah AIDS Foundation also kept track of the information in the obituaries. Robert Austin, who worked as the education director of the UAF, relied on them when "somebody wasn't returning my calls."[49] Because so many of the UAF's volunteers also had AIDS, Austin used this information to track the deaths of both volunteers and clients. Thus, obituaries proved invaluable in helping organizations working in AIDS to keep their patient censuses and volunteer lists accurate and, as a result, to allocate scarce resources appropriately.

So many of my gay narrators discussed playing AIDS "parlor games" that doing so became its own ritual of community mourning. It helped people track the scope of the epidemic at a time when other forms of news coverage remained scarce. Patty Reagan, who ran the Salt Lake AIDS Foundation, said that the obituaries made the deaths "more visible."[50] At community gatherings, gay folks swapped the names of people who had died recently, using the obituaries as one of many sources for this information. Discussing the obituaries, as hard as it was, fostered a sense of community solidarity.

Finally, reading obituaries also produced other rituals of mourning and ways of processing grief. Trish Rickers, who began working as a receptionist at the Utah AIDS Foundation in 1990, clipped obituaries as part of her job. In addition to the help it provided keeping the UAF's files up to date, she scrapbooked them for the UAF's "memorial room." The memorial room came about when a volunteer with AIDS watching Rickers carefully paste obituaries into a scrapbook said wistfully "I hope I'm not remembered in just a little book over there in the corner." Rickers thought, *"No. They deserve a place."* "And then that's when I created that room," she explained, "And before I knew it, other people were coming in and adding stuff." The room, which Rickers still maintains, has scrapbooks of photographs from UAF events and obituaries, local panels of the AIDS quilt and materials from client funerals. It also has two comfortable chairs where anyone, community member, volunteer or employee, can just sit. As Rickers describes "there's just something in there that once you sit down it's so sacred, that's comforting."[51] And people at the Utah AIDS Foundation needed comfort. As LaDonna Moore, who ran the UAF in the early 1990s remarked sadly, "the Foundation was always kind of moving through the grief. You could always feel that."[52] Thus, Rickers' responsibility for clipping obituaries evolved into a sanctuary in which staff and volunteers could sit and acknowledge their "moving through grief." It sustained people worn thin by loss, allowing brief moments of reflection before they continued the work of responding to the epidemic.

I hope that this examination of obituaries and the ways people used them in Utah, as writers and as readers, shows the importance of archiving them as sources for understanding the history of the epidemic. Obituaries contain crucial information about the ways people thought through and wrote about their experiences. When they discuss AIDS as the cause of death, they become documents that attempt a political intervention, pushing for more visibility of its terrible costs and demanding more robust response. They indicate important but otherwise unmeasurable changes in how straight people thought about kinship and the place of gay people in their families. When combined with oral histories, obituaries give us insight into how people at the heart of the epidemic coped with the grief that threatened to swamp them. Obituaries are not just notices of death. They are generative texts. At times they have even reached out from the newsprint to shape physical spaces, creating new places to mourn and to reflect on loss.

References

1. This article emerged out of a larger public humanities project that documents the AIDS epidemic in Utah. Our project includes the "Ries/Snyder Archive" and the "HIV Oral History Project," both housed in Special Collections, J. Willard Marriott Library, University of Utah, Salt Lake City, Utah (hereafter Marriott Special Collections). We have also produced a film, *Quiet Heroes*, that can be streamed for free on Amazon Prime. The research and writing of this paper were assisted by a Mellon/ACLS Scholars & Society Fellowship from the American Council of Learned Societies. Eliza McKinney, with support from the University of Utah's Undergraduate Research Opportunity Program, helped prepare the obituaries for analysis. Jeffrey Turner advised on the design of the study and ran the statistical analyses. Julia Huddleston's had a previous life as an archivist and provided crucial guidance in thinking through the ethical issues involved in placing obituaries in archival collections. As always, I am indebted to many of my colleagues in History and Gender Studies for their unflagging support. Professors Colleen McDannell, Nadja Durbach and Darius Bost provided invaluable critiques of early versions of this paper.
2. Utah Department of Health, "Total AIDS Cases Utah and United States and Reported HIV Infections for Utah," December 31, 1992, Clinic 1A Scrapbook, Volume 1, private collection.
3. Barbara Craig, "Confidences in Medical and Health Care Records from an Archive Perspective," in *Privacy & Confidentiality Perspectives: Archivists & Archival Records*, eds. Menzi Behrnd-Klodt and Peter Wosh (Chicago: Society of American Archivists, 2005), 246-256.
4. Janice Hume, *Obituaries in American Culture* (Jackson: University of Mississippi Press, 2000), 21.
5. Les Stewart obituary, 1996, Clinic 1A Scrapbook, Volume 2, private collection.
6. For discussions of families writing obituaries see Kristen Ries and Maggie Snyder (Ries speaking), interview by Elizabeth Clement, Salt Lake City, Utah, August 11, 2015, page 20, in author's possession; Richard Starley, interview by Elizabeth Clement, Salt Lake City, Utah, October 11, 2016, page 35, box 2, folder 7, HIV Oral History Project (Accn 2958), Marriott Special Collections; Ben Williams, interview by Seth Anderson, Salt Lake City, Utah, March 18, 2016, page 55, box 2, folder 10, HIV Oral History Project (Accn 2958), Marriott Special Collections; David Andreason, interview by Seth Anderson, Salt Lake City, Utah, March 22, 2016, page 46, in author's possession.
7. Hume, 23.
8. Dagmawi Woubshet, *The Calendar of Loss: Race, Sexuality, and Mourning in the Early*

Era of AIDS (Baltimore: Johns Hopkins University Press, 2015), 60.
9. Horacio Roque Ramirez, "Gay Latino Histories/Dying to Be Remembered: AIDS Obituaries, Public Memory, and the Queer Latino Archive," in *Beyond El Barrio: Everyday Life in Latina/o America*, ed. Adrian Burgos (New York: New York University Press, 2010), 103-128.
10. Corporation of the President of the Church of Jesus Christ of Latter-Day Saints, *General Handbook of Instruction*, (no city or printer, 1976), page 108.
11. Robert Austin, interviewed by Elizabeth Clement, Salt Lake City, Utah, July 19, 2016, page 8, box 1, folder 1, HIV Oral History Project (Accn 2959).
12. Hume, 141-144.
13. Woubshet, 62.
14. Woubshet, 62.
15. Woubshet, 63.
16. For Utah narrators' discussions of ACT UP, see Richard Starley, interview by Elizabeth Clement, Salt Lake City Utah, September 29, 2016, page 48 box 2, folder 7, HIV Oral History Project (Accn 2958); Kristen Ries and Maggie Snyder (Snyder speaking), interview by Elizabeth Clement, Salt Lake City, Utah, September 4, 2015, page 23, in author's possession; Ben Barr, interview by Elizabeth Clement, Point Richmond, California, April 2, 2016, page 105-6, box 1, folder 2, HIV Oral History Project (Accn 2958), Marriott Special Collections; David Andreason, interview by Seth Anderson, Salt Lake City, Utah, March 22, 2016, page 66, in author's possession.
17. Ben Williams' obituaries can be found in the Utah Pride Center Records (Accn 1918) at the University of Utah's Marriott Library, box 22, folder 3 and box 38, folder 7.
18. Snyder's obituaries are contained in her "Clinic 1A" scrapbooks. Clinic 1A Scrapbook, Volumes 1-4, Maggie Snyder Papers, private collection.
19. Corporation of the President of the Church of Jesus Christ of Latter-Day Saints, *General Handbook of Instruction*, (no city or printer, 1976), page 108.
20. Bryant Park obituary, Clinic 1A Scrapbook, Volume 1.
21. Robbie Dean Johnson obituary, Clinic 1A Scrapbook, Volume 2.
22. Roque Ramirez also combines references to AIDS as a cause of death and donations to ASOs but does not break those numbers out specifically. Roque Ramirez, 109.
23. Roque Ramirez, 109.
24. Tom Morganthau, "Gay America in Transition," *Newsweek*, August 8, 1983, 33.
25. Based on oral history estimates, which are admittedly a very fuzzy measure, between 50-70% of natal kin had some contact with men dying of AIDS and thus also met the gay kin or members of gay community organizations who

supported them.
26. Gregory Prince, *Gay Rights and the Mormon Church: Intended Actions, Unintended Consequences* (Salt Lake City: University of Utah Press, 2019), 47.
27. The oral history data indicates that gay people read "friend" or "good friend" as a reference to lover. As Don Austen said in response to my question of the meaning of the word "friend" in death rituals "sometimes in the paper they would put "and a very good friend." I clarified, "And was that seen as code," to which he responded, "Yeah. We kind of saw it as code." Don Austen, interview by Elizabeth Clement, Salt Lake City, Utah, August 23, 2017, pages 35-36, in author's possession.
28. Woubshet, 60.
29. "Stanley Marc Nelson" is an ethnically appropriate pseudonym as his obituary attributes his death to an unspecified "long illness." "Stanley Marc Nelson" obituary, Clinic 1A Scrapbook, Volume 1, private collection.
30. David Decker Freezy Frost obituary, Clinic 1A Scrapbook, Volume 1, private collection.
31. George Chauncey, "The Post-War Sex Crimes Panic," in *True Stories from the American Past*, Volume II, ed. William Graebner, third edition, (New York: McGraw Hill, 2002) 160-178; Estelle Freedman, "'Uncontrolled Desires: The Response to the Sexual Psychopath, 1920-1960," *Journal of American History*, Vol. 74, No. 1 (Jun., 1987): 83-106.
32. Steven Scott Markland obituary, Clinic 1A Scrapbook, Volume 1.
33. Les Stewart obituary, Clinic 1A Scrapbook, Volume 2, private collection.
34. Armistead Maupin, *Sure of You* (New York: Harper and Row, 1989), 85.
35. Rick Pace, interview by Elizabeth Clement, Palm Springs, California, February 13, 2016, page 9-10, box 2, folder 2, HIV Oral History Project (Accn 2958), Marriott Special Collections. For other discussions of PWA's thanking Ries without discussing AIDS in obituaries, see Ben Williams, interview by Seth Anderson, Salt Lake City, Utah, March 18, 2016, page 55, box 2, folder 10, HIV Oral History Project (Accn 2958), Marriott Special Collections.
36. Ben Williams, interview by Seth Anderson, Salt Lake City, Utah, March 18, 2016, page 55, box 2, folder 10, HIV Oral History Project (Accn 2958).
37. Patty Reagan, interview by Elizabeth Clement, Salt Lake City, June 16, 2016, page 41, , box 2, folder 3, HIV Oral History Project (Accn 2958).
38. Rick Pace, interview by Elizabeth Clement, Palm Springs, California, February 13, 2016, page 9-10, in author's possession.
39. "Thank You Dr. Kristen Ries and Maggie," *Salt Lake Tribune*, October 2, 1994, E1. For other examples of print media in Utah noting the practice of thanking Dr. Ries, see Michael Phillips, "Ministering Angel," *Salt Lake City Magazine*,

(November/December 1994): 74-80.
40. Joe Munsey, interview by Jenny Mackenzie, Salt Lake City, Utah, August 22, 2015, page 14, in author's possession.
41. Kristen Ries and Maggie Snyder, interview by Elizabeth Clement, Salt Lake City, Utah, August 11, 2015, page 22, in author's possession. For other discussions of families writing obituaries see Kristen Ries and Maggie Snyder (Ries speaking), interview by Elizabeth Clement, Salt Lake City, Utah, August 11, 2015, page 20, in author's possession; Richard Starley, interview by Elizabeth Clement, Salt Lake City, Utah, October 11, 2016, page 35, box 2, folder 7, HIV Oral History Project (Accn 2958), Marriott Special Collections.
42. Ben Williams, interview by Seth Anderson, Salt Lake City, Utah, March 18, 2016, page 51, box 2, folder 10, HIV Oral History Project (Accn 2958).
43. Amy Hoffman, *Hospital Time* (Durham: Duke University Press, 1997), 111-2.
44. David Andreason, interview by Seth Anderson, Salt Lake City, Utah, March 22, 2016, page 46, in author's possession.
45. Deborah Gould, *Moving Politics: Emotion and ACT UP's Fight Against AIDS* (Chicago: University of Chicago Press, 2009).
46. Nikki Boyer, interview by Seth Anderson, Salt Lake City Utah, June 7, 2016, page 24, in author's possession.
47. Joe Munsey, interview by Jenny Mackenzie, Salt Lake City, August 22, 2015, page 11, in author's possession. Munsey's discussion of anger inoculating him from shame supports Deborah Gould's argument that early in the epidemic gay people responded with shame, wondering if, in fact, conservative religious leaders who called AIDS "God's wrath" had a point. ACT UP, she then argues, both harnessed and transformed a growing sense of rage as the epidemic grew worse and worse, a rage that helped many people reject shame. Gould, pages 121-212.
48. Kristen Ries and Maggie Snyder (Snyder speaking), interview by Elizabeth Clement, Salt Lake City, Utah, August 11, 2015, page 21, in author's possession.
49. Robert Austin, interview by Elizabeth Clement, Salt Lake City, Utah, July 19, 2016, page 8, box 1, folder 1, HIV Oral History Project (Accn 2958), Marriott Special Collections.
50. Patty Reagan, interview by Elizabeth Clement, Salt Lake City, June 16, 2016, page 41, box 2, folder 3, HIV Oral History Project (Accn 2958), Marriott Special Collections.
51. Patricia Rickers, interview by Elizabeth Clement, Salt Lake City, September 23, 2016, page 80, box 2, folder 5, HIV Oral History Project (Accn 2958), Marriott Special Collections.
52. LaDonna Moore, interview by Elizabeth Clement, Salt Lake City, Utah, April 22, 2016, page 68, box 1, folder 10, HIV Oral History Project (Accn 2958), Marriott Special Collections.

Chapter Six

Love is Stronger than Death: Making Meaning of AIDS in the Sermons of Jim Mitulski

Lynne Gerber, PhD
Independent Scholar, San Francisco, California

Abstract

The AIDS crisis generated many religious and spiritual responses as people with AIDS and those who loved and cared for them sought to make meaning from the crisis and persevere in the face of its hardships. This paper looks at one such response by an out gay minister, the Rev. Jim Mitulski, and his LGBT congregation, the Metropolitan Community Church of San Francisco (MCCSF). Located in the Castro, San Francisco's iconic gay neighborhood and the one most impacted by AIDS, MCCSF offered a religious space for people to grapple with the meaning of AIDS in a community that affirmed the lives and relationships of gay and lesbian people. This paper examines how Rev. Mitulski used his sermons to give expression to the emotional gravitas the community was steeped in and to channel feeling toward action. It looks at how Mitulski used both canonical biblical texts and contemporary gay/lesbian literature to sacralize the experience of AIDS and make it endurable.

Religion is largely absent from the way the AIDS crisis in the United States is narrated. When addressed at all, the conversation is often limited to inflammatory statements made by Christian right leaders such as Jerry Falwell's infamous comment that AIDS was God's punishment of gay people and the societies that tolerate them (quoted in Johnson and Eskridge, 2007). The notion of AIDS as God's wrath had such cultural power – as a reflection of authentically held views about the meaning of the disease and/or as an abhorrent example of faith-based homophobia requiring rebuttal – that it was and often still dominates our understanding of the place of religion in the pre-cocktail years of the epidemic. Scholars such as Petro (2015) and Jordan (2011) have tried to map a more complex terrain, documenting the ways mainline religious groups responded to AIDS, analyzing tensions and contradictions about religion and AIDS in the writings of figures as varied as C. Everett Koop and the United States Catholic Bishops, and interpreting the explicitly religious dimensions of AIDS activism such as ACT UP's 1989 Stop the Church action.[1] This vital excavation raises even more questions about the intersection of AIDS and American religious life and what stories have been obscured by the sheer rhetorical force of "God's wrath."

Religion is also frequently absent from LGBT and San Francisco histories. San Francisco is often depicted as a secular city, a depiction that is accurate when religion is limited to participation in formal worship services and other groups (Pew 2014). Perspectives on religion that include counter-cultural spiritual practices and communities, best-selling publications in self-help and spirituality, alternative healing, and spiritual dimensions of seemingly secular social movements, suggest that San Francisco can also be seen as a source of tremendous spiritual and religious experimentation and inspiration. This becomes increasingly evident when taking a wide-angle view of religious responses to AIDS. The Shanti Project, one of the most significant AIDS support organizations in San Francisco, had spiritual roots and religious/spiritual commitments motivated some of its staff and volunteers, but the program intentionally did not talk about religion in its work. Public expressions of grief, loss and memory such as the Names Quilt, the AIDS Vigil and the annual Candlelight Marches had religious overtones and active participation from religious leaders and communities but were not explicitly religious. Relatedly, gay San Francisco is often depicted as secular. Despite the early and critical roles played by religious groups such as the Council on Religion and the Homosexual in the years before Stonewall (White 2015), many prominent gay voices from the 1980s and 90s understood gay rights and gay liberation as structurally opposed to religion (although not spirituality).[2]

This paper is part of a larger effort at telling one of those lesser-told stories, that of the Metropolitan Community Church of San Francisco (MCCSF) and its pastor of fourteen years, Reverend Jim Mitulski. It begins with basic overview of MCCSF's history and that of Reverend Mitulski. I then to turn my attention to the question of sermons and the kinds of sources they can be for historical research. Finally, I present two excepts from sermons Mitulski delivered during the height of the crisis. I will analyze his use of both canonical Christian sources paired with gay/lesbian literature to make meaning of the AIDS crisis as the congregation was living it. The sermons, I suggest, were deigned to give this community emotional and spiritual tools to endure and engage a struggle that was physically, spiritually, socially and politically unrelenting and exhausting.

This paper is drawn almost entirely from an archive of audio materials preserved by the congregation by historical accident. In 1987 the congregation began recording two of its three Sunday worship services as part of its ministry to people with AIDS. Church deacons took copies of the recording along with communion to their regular visits with house-, hospital- or hospice-bound members to keep them connected to the life of the community and the sustenance of communal worship. In 2007, when the congregation was preparing to leave its building, a long-time member noticed that someone had tagged the original recordings as garbage. They personally preserved them, removing the tapes from the bin and storing them under the raised floor in the church's sound room. They became known to me, and to church leaders, when this person learned of my research and asked if they might be of interest. The collection contains over 1,200 cassettes. With the help of a team of student researchers, I've been able to digitize and transcribe 325. The recordings document more than the sermons I'm discussing today. They include music and singing, prayers offered by clergy and people in the pews, announcements about deaths, hospitalizations, and families visiting, and greetings by many prominent visitors to the congregation. But they are especially valuable for those sermons because, for reasons outlined below, Rev. Mitulski did not keep written texts of the sermons he delivered. I mention this as a reminder that archival sources about the history of AIDS come in unexpected forms and from almost-forgotten places. Call it grace, call it luck, but this is one of those archive stories that should spur historians to keep an eye out for other unlikely sources on the verge of being permanently lost.

MCC San Francisco was the second congregation founded as part of the Universal Fellowship of Metropolitan Community Churches (UFMCC). UFMCC was founded by the Reverend Troy Perry in October of 1968, a few months before the events at Stonewall (Perry 1972, Wilcox 2003, White 2015). A holiness minister who was expelled from a number of Pentecostal congregations because of his sexual orientation, Perry came to believe that God was calling him to start a church that would welcome and minister to gays and lesbians as a legitimate – even a sacred – part of God's creation. The first meeting was held in Perry's Los Angeles living room, which rapidly grew in numbers and spurred the formation of other congregations including the one in San Francisco. A product of the moment where LGBT activism was just beginning to turn from the homophile movement to gay liberation (D'Emilio 1983), Perry's message focused on God's love for gays and lesbians and their relationships, while emphasizing that UFMCC was a Christian church, not a gay one (Perry 1972, Enroth and Jamison 1974).

The San Francisco church was founded in 1970 at Jackson's, a gay bar in North Beach. Its founder was Howard Wells, a young gay man who experienced a religious conversion of sorts at Perry's Los Angeles church meetings and wanted to form a similar community in his home city. In 1971 the congregation sponsored a revival featuring Perry that added numbers and institutional heft to the fledging church. It continued to grow throughout the 70s, meeting in different locations around the city and under the leadership of multiple pastors. In 1979 the church purchased a building at 150 Eureka Street where it stayed through the 2000s, becoming known as the pink and purple church in the Castro. At its height the congregation had over 500 members and held at least four worship services a week. One of few public spaces owned by a gay/lesbian organization, it was the site of the first public meetings about the emergence of KS, hosted hundreds of memorial services, and housed HIV support groups, 12-step addition recovery meetings, and the offices of many gay and AIDS organizations.

Jim Mitulski became the pastor of the congregation in May of 1986 when he was 27 years old. He was raised Roman Catholic in suburban Detroit where he belonged to a parish committed to the modernist reforms of Vatican II. His education and career were shaped by an overlapping set of religious, literary, and political sensibilities that he integrated in his ministry. He came out in high school, including to the clergy in his home parish who were largely supportive, and went to college at Columbia where he studied religion, read feminist and liberation theologies, and began attending the MCC congregation in New York. In the early 1980s he was part of cohort of young, progressive, out gay clergy that saw in UFMCC an opportunity to build something akin to the base communities of liberation theology for gays and lesbians. Rather than emphasize the Christian dimension of UFMCC, this group emphasized its gay/lesbian dimension and formed their liturgical and communal life with those imperatives at the forefront. Mitulski and his then-partner Bob Crocker, who became the music director of MCC San Francisco, brought these sensibilities to MCC San Francisco.

He also brought direct experience with AIDS. An associate pastor at MCC New York in the early 1980s when the disease first emerged, he was frequently called upon as a chaplain to patients with the new disease at St.

Vincent's hospital. MCC San Francisco, when they began their pastoral search process in 1986, realized that AIDS would become the center of the new minister's work. In the early years of the disease, the congregation decided its role in the epidemic was to be a place of sanctuary, providing spiritual support for people with AIDS and those working directly with them in other contexts, such as Shanti. By the mid-80s, as the scope of the disease was becoming overwhelmingly evident, church leaders started to think about ways the church could take a more active role in relation to AIDS. Mitulski's combination of progressive, feminist theology, hands-on experience with AIDS, and a gift for homiletics fit the congregation's vision of what it wanted to be in the epidemic's next stages. During his fourteen-year tenure Mitulski's preaching increasingly became a way for both he, the congregation, and the Castro community to make meaning from the crisis they were facing.

Sermons are important yet under-studied sources, especially in histories of more recent periods when other kinds of sources abound. A sermon, as traditionally understood, is religious instruction delivered in spoken form by a faith leader during a worship service. It is based on sacred literature and is used as an opportunity to help the community of listeners better understand that literature, its religious meaning and, often, its application to daily life. It is an oral genre. Although many clergy carefully compose their sermons as written texts, they are meant to be heard, not read. This is especially true of Mitulski's work. By his own account, he does not draft full texts of his sermons. Rather, in advance of preaching he gathers themes and source materials that he wishes to reflect upon and organizes some thoughts about them. But his preaching style relies upon an embodied practice of what he calls "reading the room." "I think this is why . . . I'm effective as a preacher," he said in an interview. "I'm not slick. I'm not charismatically good looking or anything like that. But I can go into a room and if there's something there that needs to be said or that wants to be expressed, by the people present, living or dead, . . . I can do it. . . . And so I prep material and then I read the room and release it. And I couldn't write it in advance if I had to." (Mitulski 2015) This approach to preaching underscores the value of an audio archive. Because he never wrote them out, we would not have a collection of Mitulski's sermons were it not for a collection of recordings from which texts could subsequently be transcribed. It also highlights the significance of the audio experience itself when it comes to spoken materials such as sermons. The sermon as a source gets its affective power not just from its content, but from its delivery. In this context the feeling quality of the delivery gives us a sense of the affective tenor of the times and the ways in which Mitulski uses affect to give shape, meaning and direction to the overwhelming emotional experience of the crisis.

A second point about sermons is their reliance on sacred text as inspiration, organizing principle, and resource for religious teaching. In the Christian tradition, sermons have typically centered on canonically recognized biblical sources and interpreted them in ways that illuminates the religious teaching the preacher is trying to convey. In Mitulski's case, he was part of a church experiment made up of mostly out, mostly faith-full (although the specifics of that faith varied significantly), gays and lesbians who were carving out an affirming space within a tradition which was deeply ambivalent at best about whether such people can be legitimate members at all. Both he and the congregation, informed by liberation theology, were committed to putting Christianity in conversation with gay experience, holding both as co-equal authorities on religious life and religious experience. He used both as resources from which to make meaning of the existential crisis at hand, meaning that did not reinscribe dominant Christian views about the sinfulness of homosexuality. He did this in two ways. First, he used canonical biblical sources to provide insight into the specific spiritual challenges of living in a time of AIDS and succor for enduring them. Second, he used gay and lesbian literature to help congregants understand what church can be for the gay/lesbian community during the AIDS crisis.

The first example is from a sermon delivered in February of 1991 after the church started sponsoring a program called AIDS and Our Relationships. It's based on second Kings chapter 2, verses 1-12, part of the prophetic literature of the Hebrew Bible. The story is of the death of the prophet Elijah and his student Elisha. It recounts how Elijah foretells his own impending death, news of which Elisha vigorously resists. After several anguished exchanges, Elijah asks Elisha what he could do for his student before they must part. Elisha, finally out of denial, makes a request. In Jim's telling, this ancient Hebrew story becomes one of immense spiritual value for a community navigating loss.

> I think the most beautiful part of the story takes place at the end where Elijah and Elisha are talking and Elisha's able to say, is able to grasp I think what's happening and he says alright, if you're going to leave I want something from you. I want a double share of your spirit to dwell in me. And Elijah says to him you want a very hard thing, but there's one way for you to have this if you want it. And that's to be with me through this. That's the only way that you'll get a thing that you want. He says if you, if you, if you stay with me, if you see me as I am being taken from you it shall be so for you. One

thing that gives me hope in this midst of AIDS and our relationships is this. We can't control the outcome; we are not in control. We have to let go, let go, let go, always letting go. But if we're able to be there for each other and with each other, whoever we are in this constellation -- a person with HIV, not a person with HIV, several people with HIV, people with not -- if we're able to see it through with each other, that's all that we can hope for and that's where we find the blessing. That's where we get the double share of spirit, whatever it means. Sticking through it, sticking together, being together. That's how we inherit the double portion of spirit that Elisha coveted (Mitulski 1991a).

This clip shows a very different approach to the intersection of religion and AIDS. Mitulski does not attempt to find meaning in AIDS by trying to decipher God's intention in the disease, the timing of its appearance, or the people it afflicts. Rather, he uses scriptural sources to explicate the importance of staying with each other through pain and loss and to suggest that doing so generates real spiritual gifts – double blessings – for those who can do so. He counters the message of the right by looking for the blessing that can be found in AIDS, not the curse. Iit is not an easy blessing; these are not sermons of religious platitudes. Rather, they use biblical texts to find and cultivate the spiritual resources needed to be able to stay together, to stay with each other through the horrors of illness and the pain of loss. Scripture is not used to deny or obfuscate the difficulties of sticking it through; in other sermons on this text he acknowledges that people can't always do it, especially people like those in this community who are asked to do it again and again and again (Mitulski 1995). Rather it is used as living text that can provide sustenance for people that may be grasping for ways to sit with one more person, with one more loss, for one more day.

The second example is from a sermon delivered later that year in November. In this case, Mitulski draws upon imagery by lesbian poet Adrienne Rich (1983) to imagine what church can and should be for people facing these kinds of losses. The sermon is a reflection on a feeling Mitulski was experiencing himself and saw in the congregation –being tired of people dying. At the time San Francisco was still climbing toward its peak number of AIDS deaths in 1992. The magnitude and relentlessness of loss was overwhelming and the community was exhausted. But church, he said, was and should be a place where people could bring that tiredness and its vast attendant feelings for a measure of relief and transformation into action. He said:

There's no answer to this feeling of what to do when we're sick of people dying. And yet I know the most important thing that we can do, the thing that's within our control, is to find ways for us all to express the depth of our sorrow, and our grief, and our anger, and our numbness, and our tears, and our laughter too when that's appropriate. That's the best gift we can give each other at this time. The lesbian poet Adrienne Rich says in one of her poems, "there must be those among whom we can weep and still be counted as warriors." The church, and communities like it, are places like that. A place where we can come together, where we can weep, and where people will still recognize that we are warriors. I don't know that I like the imagery necessarily of a fight or war against AIDS, and yet this is, that's how it feels sometimes. And it's not a fight I want to lose or that I'm willing gently to let one more person be lost into. Expressing our feelings is the one thing that we can do, and channeling it into action is something else that we can do. Demonstrations, political action, supporting the community, giving money. These are all ways, small ways, that we have of breaking out of the paralysis that can take place in us when we feel that we're sick of people dying. We can't stop people from dying. Every one of us will die, I know we know that. We say it a lot, it's one of those things we say to comfort ourselves, I don't know why we say it, but it does, it's true. All of us face that. Some of us have HIV, some of us don't. None of us want to die, it seems. But this is a place where we can still come together, week after week after week, and weep and still be counted as warriors. A place where our relationships can continue to flourish. A place where we can still continue to know love and to live life fully as long as we have it, until it's over, and even then, I'm not sure it's ever over (Mitulski 1991b).

In this excerpt Mitulski uses Rich's imagery to help the congregation recognize its own sorrows as both a sign *of* and a resource *for* struggles worth engaging in – for GLBT acceptance, for a cure, and for keeping an open, tender heart in the middle of pain and loss. Gay/lesbian cultural resources, in the form of Rich's work, is sacralized by its centrality in the sermon and is used to focus attention on the glint of the sacred in gay life and gay culture. He then uses it to show that the church can house and cultivate that sacred. He does so not just in the sermon's content, but in the emotional transparency of its delivery. Mitulski is reflecting the tiredness and uncertainty of his community here, but in acknowledging it with such candor, by naming it as sacred, he's able to move the congregation to a place past those feelings, a place where weeping is both true and not the end of the story. Weeping, in this sermon, is as real, ever-present and exhausting as it was felt by many congregants, but is also becomes a sign of battle, of engaging faithfully in a good fight, a fight that in 1991 seemed far from over.

There's a great deal that can be learned from recordings such as these and sermons such as Mitulski's. In them we hear of how national moments and events play out in a micro-context such as when Mitulski preaches on the 1987 and the 1993 Marches on Washington. We can trace some of the affective trajectory of the epidemic as we listen week after week as preachers try to make spiritual and emotional sense of the circumstances they were living through. And we can hear how religion was used in the crisis not to condemn but to give strength to those who were sick, grieving, caring, and dying. They are an example of a religious community that was able to make meaningful use of canonical scripture in a crisis in part because it already resolved for itself the question of if or how LGBT people fit in the tradition and insisted not only on their rightful place in it but the importance of their contributions to it; contributions that included their response to AIDS. The case of MCC San Francisco and Jim Mitulski's sermons undercuts the notion that religious and gay communities were irreconcilable and that religious communities in San Francisco were either absent from the epidemic or hamstrung by theological contradictions about those who were disproportionately affected by it. Mitulski's sermons show us how a community of faith insisted that their struggles with AIDS and the socio-political context in which they were forged were not only not meaningless, but were able to give new meaning to a tradition that in so many other contexts fell silent in the face of AIDS.

Endnotes

1. For other discussions of AIDS and/in American religious life in the pre-cocktail years see Jordan, 2011, Mumford 2016, O'Loughlin 2019, Royles 2020.
2. For a contemporary example see Jones 1985a, 1985b and 1985c. For reflections on the limitations of historiographic framing of religion and sexuality more generally, as well as an articulation of new possibilities, see Frank, Moreton and White 2018.

References

D'Emilio, J. (1983). *Sexual politics, sexual communities*. University of Chicago.

Enroth, R. M. and Jamison, G. E. (1974). *The gay church*. Eerdmans.

Frank, G., Moreton, B., and White, H.R. (2018). Introduction: More than missionary: Doing the histories of religion and sexuality together. In G. Frank, B. Moreton and H. R. White eds. *Devotions and desires: Histories of sexuality and religion in the twentieth-century United States* (pp. 1-16). University of North Carolina.

Johnson, H. and Eskridge, W. (2007, May 19). The legacy of Falwell's bully pulpit. *Washington Post*, A17. https://www.washingtonpost.com/wpdyn/content/article/2007/05/18/AR2007051801392.html

Jones, B. (1985a, April 25). The church and us, Part one. *Bay Area Reporter* 15(17), 6.

Jones, B. (1985b, May 2). The church and us, Part two. *Bay Area Reporter* 15(18), 6.

Jones, B. (1985c, May 9). The church and us, Part three. *Bay Area Reporter* 15(19), 6

Jordan, M. D. (2011). *Recruiting young love: How Christians talk about homosexuality*. University of Chicago Press.

Mitulski, J. (1991a, February 10). Untitled sermon. Metropolitan Community Church of San Francisco Archives. San Francisco, California. Transcript in possession of the author.

Mitulski, J. (1991b, November 17). Untitled sermon. Metropolitan Community Church of San Francisco Archives. San Francisco, California. Transcript in possession of the author.

Mitulski, J. (1995, August 6). Untitled sermon. Metropolitan Community Church of San Francisco Archives. San Francisco, California. Transcript in possession of the author.

Mitulski, J. (2015, July 29). Personal interview with L. Gerber and M. D. Jordan. San Francisco, California.

Mumford, K. J. (2016). *Not straight, not white: Black gay men from the march on Washington to the AIDS crisis*. University of North Carolina.

Perry, T. (1972). *The lord is my shepherd and he knows I'm gay*. Nash.

Petro, A. (2016). *After the wrath of God: AIDS, sexuality and American religion*. Oxford University.

Pew Research Center (2014). Adults in the San Francisco Metro Area. Religious Landscapes Study. https://www.pewforum.org/religious-

landscape-study/metro-area/san-francisco-metro-area/
Rich, A. (1983). *Sources*. Heyeck.
Royles, D. (2020). *To make the wounded whole: The African American struggle against HIV/AIDS*. University of North Carolina.
O'Loughlin, M. (Producer). (2019-2020). Plague: Untold stories of AIDS and the Catholic church [Podcast]. *America Media*. https://www.americamagazine.org/plague
White, H. (2015). *Reforming Sodom: Protestants and the rise of gay rights*. University of North Carolina.
Wilcox, M. (2003). *Coming out in Christianity: Religion, identity and community*. Indiana University.

Index

Abrams, Donald L., 1, 3–5, 7, 14
ACT UP, 60, 80–83, 89–90, 95*n*47, 97
African Americans, 76–77
African swine fever virus, 7
AIDS: ARV, 14, 16, 18; cancer and, 87–88; as "God's wrath," 95*n*47, 96–97; oral lesion as early sign of, 19; pandemic, 68; patients, white blood cells from, 12–13; virus, 7–9, 12–19, 22. *See also* HIV; *specific topics*
AIDS and Our Relationships program, of MCCSF, 101
AIDS Clinic, at SFGH, 9, 68
AIDS crisis, religion and spirituality in response to, 96–104
AIDS epidemic: contact tracing and, 28; daily experience of, 90; obituaries and, 76–77, 80–82, 90–91; oral history of, 72–74; in San Francisco, 68, 72–74, 102; in Utah, 76–77, 90
The AIDS Epidemic in San Francisco (Hughes), 68
AIDS obituaries: AIDS epidemic and, 76–77, 80–82, 90–91; four framing categories of, 78; homosexuality in, 79–80, 82–87; kinship sentence of, 78, 83–87; Latinx, 79; in mainstream newspapers *versus* gay newspapers, 78–84; Maupin on, 87–89; in 1980s and 1990s, 79–80; Ries mentioned in, 88; from Snyder collection, 81–82, 84–86; in Utah, 76–91; from Williams collection, 81–89
AIDS Program, Yale School of Medicine, 56
AIDS Service Organization (ASO), 82
AIDS-associated Retroviruses (ARV), 14, 16, 18
Ammann, Art, 9–10
Andreason, David, 89–90
Annals of Internal Medicine, 17
anthropology, HIV and, 51–53, 56, 58
antibodies, to HIV, 20–21
Arnstein, Paul, 13–14
ARV. *See* AIDS-associated Retroviruses
ASO. *See* AIDS Service Organization
Austen, Don, 94*n*27
Austin, Robert, 90

Baehr v. Lewin, 85
BAR. *See Bay Area Reporter*
Barnes, David, 70
Barré-Sinoussi, Francoise, 12
basic research, in HIV/AIDS, 3
Bay Area Reporter (*BAR*), 79, 83–84
The Berkeley Remix podcast, 72–73

Bibace, R., 54
biblical texts, in Mitulski sermons, 96, 101–2
Biogard Biosafety Hood, 5–6
biosafety hoods, 5–7, 11, 13
Bishop, Mike, 12
Black men and Black women, HIV and, 55
blood donors, HIV contamination and, 28, 32, 34
Bloom's taxonomy, 56–57
Boyer, Nikki, 90
Brabant, S., 52
Brown, P. J., 54
Brown, Willie, 9–11
Burkitt lymphoma patients, 20
Bush, Barbara, 80
Bush, George H. W., 80

CAF. *See* cell antiviral factor
California History-Social Science Project, 72
Calisphere, 68, 71
the Castro, San Francisco, 96, 99–100
CD4+ cells, 12, 19, 21
CD8+ cells, 21–22
CDC. *See* Centers for Disease Control and Prevention
cell antiviral factor (CAF), 21–22
Centers for Disease Control and Prevention (CDC), 31, 55, 58
Chermann, Jean-Claude, 12
Chiron, 15
The Church of Jesus Christ of Latter-day Saints. *See* Mormon Church
Clavel, Francois, 12
"Clip and Mail AIDS Obits" campaign, of ACT UP, 80–81
CMV, 8

CNAR, 22
coming out, gay community on, 80, 83–84
Common Core State Standards, 71
Conant, Marcus, 5–7, 9
contact tracing: in AIDS epidemic, arguments against, 28; approaches to, 26–28; confidentiality, autonomy and, 33, 35–36; definitions, 27; for epidemics and pandemics, 26, 35–36; history of, 26; partner notification in, 27–28, 30–32; for STIs, 26, 34; voluntary *versus* mandatory, 33
contact tracing, for HIV, 25; GBV and, 30–31; HIV testing and, 28, 30, 35; legal and ethical issues, 31–34; mandatory, in New York, 32; partner notification in, 30–31, 35; social and cultural considerations, 35; STIs and, 30, 34–36; universal, 28–30, 35–37
Contagious Diseases Acts of 1864, 26
coronavirus, 5
Council on Religion and the Homosexual, 97
COVID-19 pandemic, 2–3, 22, 25, 62, 70
Craik, Charlie, 16
criminalization, of HIV, 32–33, 57, 60
Crocker, Bob, 99
Cutter Laboratories, 19
cytopathic effects, of HIV, 13

Deseret News, 79
Dirksen, Ellen, 8–9
DNA restriction enzyme patterns, 16–17
Dominican Republic (DR), 7
Drew, Larry, 8
Dritz, Selma, 7

drug use, HIV and, 53, 61, 81
"Drugs, Sex, and HIV" course, 49, 56–60, 62

EBV. *See* Epstein-Barr virus
electron microscopic (EM), 4–5, 14
ELISA. *See* enzyme linked immunoassay
EM. *See* electron microscopic
enzyme linked immunoassay (ELISA), 28
"Epidemics in History" curriculum, 67
epidemiology, of HIV, 52–53, 57, 60–61
Epstein, Steve, 70
Epstein-Barr virus (EBV), 19–20
ethnography, HIV and, 52–53, 58

faith-based homophobia, 96–97
Falwell, Jerry, 96
FDA. *See* Food and Drug Administration
Fieldsteel, Howard, 13–14
First Response podcast, 70, 73
Florida, HIV in, 55–56
Florida Department of Health, 55
Food and Drug Administration (FDA), 28, 58
Frost, David Decker Freezy, 86

Gallo, Bob, 12, 16–20
Gallup, 83–84
Gandhi, Monica, 1
Gardner, Murray, 9–10, 16–17
gay community, 7, 28, 72–73, 77, 80–84, 88–91, 101
gay liberation, 80, 97–99
gay marriage, 85
gay men: HIV and, 51–52, 61; KS and, 4; Latinx, obituaries, in San Francisco, 79; obituaries of, Williams collection, 82; in San Francisco, Maupin on, 87–89; white, in Utah, 76
gay newspapers, 79–84
Gay Related Immune Deficiency (GRID), 5, 7–8
gay rights, 97
gay/lesbian literature, 96–98, 101
Gazdar, Adi, 20
GBV. *See* gender-based violence
Gen Z and Millennials, HIV education for, 53–56, 61
gender-based violence (GBV), 30–31, 34
The General Handbook of Instruction, of Mormon Church, 79, 82
Gould, Deborah, 89–90, 95n47
Greenspan, Deborah, 20
Greenspan, John, 9–10, 20
GRID. *See* Gay Related Immune Deficiency

HAART. *See* highly active antiretroviral therapy
Hackett, Adeline, 13–14
Haiti, AIDS and, 7–8
Hartley, Janet, 17
health care access, HIV infection and, 33, 50
Health Insurance Portability and Accountability Act of 1996 (HIPAA), 77
hemophiliacs, 19, 22, 81
Henle, Gertrude, 19–20
Henle, Werner, 19–20
hepatitis B, 8
hepatitis C, 53
herpesvirus, 4–5, 21
heterosexual sex, HIV and, 52
HHV-8, 4
highly active antiretroviral therapy

(HAART), 30
HIPAA. *See* Health Insurance Portability and Accountability Act of 1996
Hispanic/Latino men, HIV and, 55
Hispaniola, 7–8
HIV: contact tracing for, 25, 28–37; exceptionalism, 50, 54; pandemic, 25, 28, 30, 35–36, 50, 57; replication, 16–18, 21; testing, 28, 30–31, 35; undergraduate college courses on, 49–62; undergraduate students and, 49, 52–56, 58–62; white blood cells and, 20–21. *See also specific topics*
HIV counseling, US Public Health Service guidelines on, 30
HIV epidemic: anthropologists on, 53; contact tracing for, 25, 35, 37; in Florida, 55; oral history of, 72
HIV transmission, 18–19, 30; criminalizing, 32–33; HAART for preventing, 30; legal and ethical requirement to prevent, 32; rape and, 33; through shared needles, 53
HIV/AIDS oral history archive, 67–74
HIV-infected cells, 18–19
Hoffman, Amy, 89
homophobia, 51, 89, 96–97
homosexuality, in AIDS obituaries, 79–80, 82–87
Hospital Time (Hoffman), 89
HTLV, 12, 14, 19
HTLV-III, 14, 16–18
Hughes, Sally Smith, 68, 72–74
human rights, 54, 61
Human Tumor Virus room, UCSF, 11
Hume, Janice, 78
HUT 78 T cell line, 20

IFA. *See* immunofluorescence antibody test
Ilieva, Polina, 3
Illinois Confidentiality of HIV-Related Information Act of 2015, 32
immune deficiency disorders, 7, 19
immune system disorders, GRID, 5
immunofluorescence antibody (IFA) test, 20
International AIDS Conference, 1996, 30

Jacob, François, 12
Jacobs, Paul, 80
Johnson, Robert Dean, 83
Jordan, M. D., 97

Kaminsky, Larry, 20–21
Kaposi's sarcoma (KS), 4–5, 7–9, 99
Kim, Young, 13–14
Koenig, Ellen, 7
Koop, C. Everett, 97
KS. *See* Kaposi's sarcoma

The Lancet, 7
Latinx folks, 76–77, 79
LAV retrovirus, 12, 14, 16–18
Lennette, Evelyne, 20
lentiviruses, 14
Levy, Jay A., 1
LGBT health care, teaching HIV and, 51–52
LGBT people, 55
LGBTQ+ communities, 68
lymphoma, 20

major symptoms, of AIDS, 5
Marches on Washington, 1987 and 1993, 104
Markland, Steven Scott, 87

Martin, Mal, 17
Maupin, Armistead, 87–89
MCCSF. *See* Metropolitan Community Church of San Francisco
Medicaid, Florida and, 55
Merck, 54–55
Metropolitan Community Church of San Francisco (MCCSF), 96–97, 99–104
migrant workers, 57
Millennials and Gen Z, HIV education for, 53–56, 61
Mitulski, Jim, 96–104
mononucleosis, 19–20
Montagnier, Luc, 12, 16, 18
Moore, LaDonna, 91
Mormon Church, 79, 82
Moss, Andrew, 7
mouse retrovirus, 13, 19
Moving Politics (Gould), 89–90
Munsey, Joe, 90, 95*n*47

Naiman, Eleanor, 74
National Endowment for the Humanities, 1
National Institutes of Health (NIH), 4, 8–9, 14–19
National Science Foundation, 8–9
Nelson, Stanley Dee, 86
Nelson-Reese, Walter, 13–14
New York Native, 80
New York Public Library, 77
New York State Archives, 77
New York Times, 80
NIH. *See* National Institutes of Health

obituaries. *See* AIDS obituaries
OHMS. *See* Oral History Metadata Synchronizer

opt out HIV testing, 28
oral history: of AIDS epidemic, 72–74; in pedagogy, 67, 69
Oral History Center at UC Berkeley and UCSF, 67–75
Oral History Metadata Synchronizer (OHMS), 71, 73–74
oral lesions, 19
Oshiro, Lyndon, 13–14

Pace, Rick, 88
pandemics, teaching during, 62
Park, Bryant, 82
Parker, R., 53
Parran, Thomas, 26, 34
partner notification, in contact tracing, 27–28, 30–32, 35
Pasteur Institute, 11–12
patient referral, in contact tracing, 27
pedagogy: about HIV, 50–51; oral history in, 67, 69; trauma-informed, 61. *See also* undergraduate college courses, on HIV
penicillin, 26
people living with AIDS (PLWA), 1–2, 55
people living with HIV, 50, 52, 56, 60–61
Perry, Troy, 98–99
Peterlin, Matija, 16
Petro, A., 97
Pillar, 81–82
PLWA. *See* People Living with AIDS
PrEP, 58
Prevention Access Campaign, 54–55
provider referral, in contact tracing, 27, 32
Prusiner, Stan, 9
Public Health Service, US, 30

Ramirez, Horacio Roque, 79, 83–84
rape, HIV infection and, 33
Rauscher, Frank, 8
Reagan, Patty, 88, 90
Reagan, Ronald, 8–9, 61
Reichman, Michelle, 8
religion and spirituality, in response to AIDS crisis, 96–104
retroviruses: ARV, 14, 16, 18; CAF and, 21; hemophiliacs and, 19; LAV, 12, 14, 16–18; mouse, 13, 19; tumors and, 13–14
reverse transcriptase (RT), 16
Rich, Adrienne, 102–4
Rickers, Trish, 91
Ries, Kristen, 81, 88
Ries/Snyder HIV Archive, at University of Utah, 77–78
Riggs, John, 13–14
Rosenberg, Charles, 70
RT. *See* reverse transcriptase
Rutter, Bill, 15
Rwandan genocide, 33

Salhi, B. A., 54
Salt Lake City, 80–82, 88
Salt Lake Tribune, 79, 81–82, 88
San Francisco: AIDS epidemic in, 68, 72–74, 102; AIDS patients in, 13; AIDS virus in, 14–15; *BAR* in, 79, 83–84; the Castro, 96, 99–100; gay community in, 1970s, 72–73; gay men in, Maupin on, 87–89; MCCSF, 96–97, 99–104; religion in, 96–97
San Francisco Chronicle, 5, 83
San Francisco General Hospital (SFGH), 4–5, 9, 13, 68
San Francisco Model, for AIDS care, 68

Science, 12, 14, 19
sermons, by Mitulski, 96–98, 100–104
sex workers, 57, 61
sexual partners, notified in contact tracing, 27–28, 30–32
sexually-transmitted infections (STIs), 25–26, 30, 33–36, 54–55
SFGH. *See* San Francisco General Hospital
Shadow on the Land: Syphilis (Parran), 26
Shanti Project, 97, 100
shared needles, HIV transmission through, 53
Smith, Helene, 13–14
Snyder, Maggie, 81–82, 84–86, 88–90
social media, 27–28, 53, 57, 61
sociology, HIV and, 51
Stampfer, Martha, 13–14
Stewart, Les, 78, 87
STIs. *See* sexually-transmitted infections
Stites, Dan, 9–10
Stonewall uprising, 1969, 79–80, 83, 97–98
Stop the Church action, of ACT UP, 1989, 97
storytelling, in history and social-studies curricula, 67–68
Sure of You (Maupin), 87–89
Sustainable Development Goals, UN, 57
syphilis, 26, 34–35

Tarasoff vs the Regents of the University of California, 32
Teas, Jane, 7
témoignage, 53
Tomes, Nancy, 70
transphobia, 51
trauma-informed pedagogy, 61
tumors, 4–5, 13–14

Tuskegee experiments, 26

UAF. *See* Utah AIDS Foundation
UCSF. *See* University of California, San Francisco
UFMCC. *See* Universal Fellowship of Metropolitan Community Churches
Uhrlich, David, 3
ultracentrifuge, to obtain HIV from culture fluids, 10, 12
UNAIDS, 57–58
undergraduate college courses, on HIV, 50–52; Bloom's taxonomy for designing goals of, 56–57; "Drugs, Sex, and HIV," 49, 56–60, 62; in Florida, 55–56; for Millennials and Gen Z, 53–55, 61
undergraduate students, HIV and, 49, 52–56, 58–62
United Nations Sustainable Development Goals, 57
United States Catholic Bishops, 97
universal contact tracing, for HIV, 28–30, 35–37
Universal Fellowship of Metropolitan Community Churches (UFMCC), 98–99
University of California, San Francisco (UCSF): AIDS researchers at, 3, 8, 11–13, 15–16; Archives & Special Collections, 1–3, 68; Conant at, 5–7; Human Tumor Virus room, 11; Oral History Center at UC Berkeley and, 67–75
University of California Berkeley, 67–75
University of Utah, 77–78
Utah: AIDS epidemic in, 76–77, 90; AIDS obituaries in, 76–91; Mormon Church in, 79, 82; Salt Lake City, 80–82, 88; white gay men in, 76
Utah AIDS Foundation (UAF), 78, 80, 82, 90–91

vaccine, for HIV/AIDS, 3, 22, 50
Venereal Diseases Control and Prevention Act of 1938, 26
viruses: AIDS, 7–9, 12–19, 22; cancer and, 5, 12–13; tumors and, 4–5, 13–14. *See also* retroviruses
Volberding, Paul A., 1, 3–4, 9–10

Walsh, M. E., 54
Weiss, Robin, 14
Weitz, Rose, 52, 56
Wells, Howard, 99
white blood cells, 12–13, 20–21
white gay men, in Utah, 76
WHO. *See* World Health Organization
Wilbur, Judy, 20
Williams, Ben, 81–89
women, HIV and, 51–52, 55, 74
Women's Prison Association (WPA), 77
World Health Organization (WHO), 33, 55, 58
Woubshet, Dagmawi, 80
WPA. *See* Women's Prison Association

Yale School of Medicine, AIDS Program, 56

zidovudine, in HIV infection treatment, 30
Ziegler, John, 9–10

www.ingramcontent.com/pod-product-compliance
Lightning Source LLC
Chambersburg PA
CBHW070654220526
45466CB00001B/441